RESEARCH REPORT

Measuring Success in Health Care Value-Based Purchasing Programs

Summary and Recommendations

Cheryl L. Damberg • *Melony E. Sorbero* • *Susan L. Lovejoy*

Grant Martsolf • *Laura Raaen* • *Daniel Mandel*

Sponsored by the Office of the Assistant Secretary for Planning and Evaluation

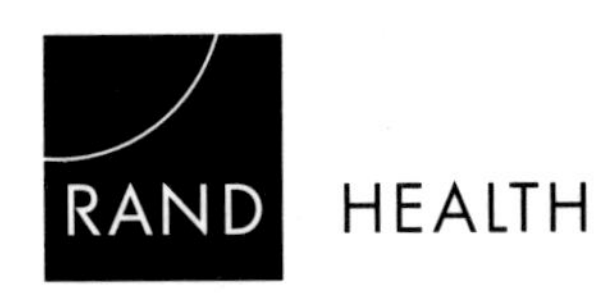

HEALTH

The research described in this report was sponsored by the Office of the Assistant Secretary for Planning and Evaluation in the U.S. Department of Health and Human Services, and was produced within RAND Health, a division of the RAND Corporation.

Library of Congress Control Number: 2013957550

ISBN 978-0-8330-8395-1

RAND OFFICES

SANTA MONICA, CA • WASHINGTON, DC

PITTSBURGH, PA • NEW ORLEANS, LA • JACKSON, MS • BOSTON, MA

CAMBRIDGE, UK • BRUSSELS, BE

Preface

The U.S. Department of Health and Human Services (HHS) is advancing the implementation of value-based purchasing (VBP) across an array of health care settings in the Medicare program in response to requirements in the 2010 Patient Protection and Affordable Care Act. VBP refers to a broad set of performance-based payment strategies that link financial incentives to providers' performance on a set of defined measures in an effort to achieve better value by driving improvements in quality and slowing the growth in health care spending. Policymakers are grappling with many policy decisions about how best to design and implement VBP programs so that they are successful in achieving stated goals.

To inform future policymaking by HHS regarding the implementation and expansion of VBP in the Medicare program, the Office of the Assistant Secretary for Planning and Evaluation (ASPE) in the HHS asked RAND to review what has been learned over the past decade with performance-based payment models (otherwise referred to as VBP). As part of the review, RAND was asked to review the elements of successful VBP programs and to identify gaps in the knowledge base that, if addressed, could improve the design and functioning of VBP programs moving forward. Three types of VBP programs were the focus of the review: (1) pay-for-performance programs, (2) accountable care organizations, and (3) bundled payments.

This report summarizes the current state of knowledge based on a review of the published literature, a review of publicly available documentation from actual VBP programs, and discussions with an expert panel composed of VBP program sponsors (i.e., health plans, community collaboratives, and public payers), providers and health systems, and academic researchers with VBP evaluation expertise. Based on this review, we outline a set of recommendations regarding the design, implementation, and monitoring and evaluation of these programs, which if pursued could help policymakers better understand where and under what conditions VBP works and how to strengthen program design and implementation so that these programs achieve improved value for patients and for payers.

The contents of this report will be of interest to public and private payers of health care who sponsor VBP programs, health care providers, policymakers, and health researchers who work to build the evidence base.

This work was sponsored by ASPE, under contract No. 12-233-SOL-00418. The work was conducted in RAND Health, a division of the RAND Corporation. A profile of RAND Health, abstracts of its publications, and ordering information can be found at www.rand.org/health.

Contents

Figure and Tables

Figure

Tables

Acknowledgments

The authors would like to thank Stephanie Glier (project officer), Dr. William Borden, and Dr. Lok Wong Samson from the Office of Health Policy within the Office of the Assistant Secretary for Planning and Evaluation (ASPE) for their valuable guidance and feedback throughout the project. We also thank Nancy De Lew and Dr. Pierre Yong of ASPE, Drs. Timothy Cuerdon and Jordan VanLare of the Centers for Medicare and Medicaid Services (CMS), and Drs. Richard Kronick and Irene Fraser of the Agency for Healthcare Research and Quality (AHRQ) for their insightful comments during the meetings of the technical expert panel and their thoughtful reviews of this report.

We are especially indebted to our expert panelists, who gave generously of their time to participate in panel discussions. These individuals graciously shared the lessons they have learned on the "front line" as VBP program designers and implementers, as providers who have had to respond to VBP programs, and as VBP program evaluators.

We also thank Drs. Jon Christianson (University of Minnesota) and Richard C. Neu (RAND) for their careful review and comments on the draft of this report, contributions that strengthen the final product.

ASPE Measuring Success in Value-Based Purchasing Technical Expert Panel	
Adams Dudley, MD, PhD University of California at San Francisco	Andrew Ryan, PhD Weill Cornell Medical College
Patrick Falvey, PhD Aurora Health Care	Dana Safran, PhD Blue Cross Blue Shield of Massachusetts
Tammy Fisher Partnership HealthPlan of California	Barbara Walters, MD Dartmouth-Hitchcock
John Hirshleifer, MD Blue Shield of California	Rachel Werner, MD, PhD ASPE and University of Pennsylvania
Elizabeth Mort, MD Partners HealthCare, Inc.	Tom Williams, DrPH and Dolores Yanagihara Integrated Healthcare Association

We also acknowledge the contributions of the following federal participants who provided the public payer perspective during the discussions of the Technical Expert Panel: Elizabeth Goldstein (CMS, Consumer Assessment and Plan Performance), John Pilotte (CMS, Performance-based Payment Policy Group), James Poyer (CMS, Division of Value, Incentives, and Quality Reporting), and Mark Wynn (CMS).

We thank Drs. Jon Christianson (University of Minnesota) and Richard C. Neu (RAND) for their careful review and comments on the draft of this report, contributions that strengthen the final product. We also acknowledge the important role played by RAND team members

Roberta Shanman, Margaret Maglione, and Lynn Polite, who provided research assistance, helped with review of the literature, and provided project support.

Abbreviations

ACA	Patient Protection and Affordable Care Act
ACO	accountable care organization
AQC	Alternative Quality Contract
ASPE	Assistant Secretary for Planning and Evaluation
CMS	Centers for Medicare and Medicaid Services
DRG	diagnostic-related group
DSH	disproportionate share hospital
ED	emergency department
EHR	electronic health record
HAC	healthcare acquired condition
HbA1c	glycated hemoglobin
HEDIS	Healthcare Effectiveness Data and Information Set
HHS	U.S. Department of Health and Human Services
HIT	health information technology
HQID	Hospital Quality Incentive demonstration
HVBP	Hospital Value-Based Purchasing Program
P4P	pay-for-performance
PROMs	Patient-Reported Outcome Measures
PVPM	Physician Value-Based Payment Modifier
SES	socioeconomic status
TEP	technical expert panel
VBP	value-based purchasing

CHAPTER ONE

Introduction

Value-based purchasing (VBP) refers to a broad set of performance-based payment strategies that link financial incentives to providers' performance on a set of defined measures. Both public and private payers are using VBP strategies in an effort to drive improvements in quality and to slow the growth in health care spending. Nearly ten years ago, the U.S. Department of Health and Human Services (HHS) and the Centers for Medicare and Medicaid Services (CMS) began testing VBP models with their hospital pay-for-performance (P4P) demonstrations, known as the Premier Hospital Quality Incentive Demonstration (HQID) and the Physician Group Practice (PGP) Demonstration, which provided financial incentives to physician groups that performed well on quality and cost metrics. The use of financial incentives as a strategy to drive improvements in care dates back even further among private payers and Medicaid programs, which began experimenting with P4P in the mid-1990s and early 2000s.[112] These early private payer P4P programs generally focused on holding providers accountable for their quality performance and targeted physician groups, individual physicians, and hospitals.[1–3]

Although the published evidence from P4P programs implemented by private-sector payers between 2000 and 2010 showed mostly modest results in improving performance,[4–11] public and private payers have continued to experiment with the use of financial incentives as a policy lever to drive improvements in care. Many of the early P4P program designs have evolved over time to include a larger and broader set of measures, including resource use and cost metrics, in an effort to reward providers for delivering value,[*] and many programs are deploying a wider range of incentives. Additionally, other VBP models have since emerged and are currently being tested, including accountable care organizations (ACOs) and bundled payment programs, which target both quality and cost.

We define each of the three broad types of VBP models as follows:

- **Pay-for-performance** refers to a payment arrangement in which providers are rewarded (bonuses) or penalized (reductions in payments) based on meeting preestablished targets or benchmarks for measures of quality and/or efficiency. Financial incentives are used to change provider behavior to achieve a set of objectives specified by the payer.
- **Accountable care organization** refers to a health care organization comprised of doctors, hospitals, and other health care providers, who voluntarily come together to provide coordinated care and agree to be held accountable for the overall costs and quality of care

[*] Value is defined as the outcomes (outputs) achieved divided by the cost or resources used (inputs) to generate those outcomes.

for an assigned population of patients. The ACO payment model ties provider reimbursements to performance on quality measures and reductions in the total cost of care. Under an ACO arrangement, providers in the ACO agree to take financial risk and are eligible for a share of the savings achieved through improved care delivery provided they achieve quality and spending targets negotiated between the ACO and the payer.

- **Bundled payments**[*] is a method in which payments to health care providers are based on the expected costs for a clinically defined episode or bundle of related health care services. The payment arrangement includes financial and quality performance accountability for the episode of care. Episodes can be defined in different ways, cover varying periods of time (e.g., one year for a chronic condition, the period of the hospital stay and 30 days post-discharge), and include single or multiple health care providers of different types (e.g., hospital only, hospital and ambulatory provider).[12–14] In this project, we limited our examination of bundled payment arrangements to those that included both cost and quality performance components to assess value.

The Medicare program has gradually been moving toward implementing VBP across various care settings starting with pay-for-reporting programs (e.g., the Hospital Inpatient Quality Reporting program and the Physician Quality Reporting Initiative) and P4P demonstrations to gain experience. The 2010 Patient Protection and Affordable Care Act (ACA)[15] significantly expands VBP by requiring the Medicare program to implement, develop plans for, and test in the context of demonstrations the use of VBP across a broad set of providers and settings of care (i.e., physicians, skilled nursing homes, home health agencies, ambulatory surgery centers, long-term hospitals, rehabilitation hospitals, cancer hospitals, psychiatric hospitals, and hospice facilities), as shown in Table 1. For example, the ACA required HHS to submit plans for implementing VBP in ambulatory surgery centers, home health agencies, and skilled nursing homes to Congress in 2011. The Hospital Value-Based Purchasing program, which features payment adjustments (both bonuses and penalties) to hospitals for performance, began implementation in October 2012, and the Physician Value-based Payment Modifier (PVPM) is slated to start in January 2015. The ACA further links provider payments to cost reductions and quality improvements through the implementation and testing of VBP models such as ACOs and bundled payments. To that end, Medicare has begun the Bundled Payments for Care Improvement demonstrations and the ACO shared savings programs and demonstrations. Moreover, Congress is actively considering ways to revise the physician fee schedule (i.e., the sustainable growth rate) to incorporate VBP incentives so that payment policy for physicians paid under fee-for-service supports the delivery of high quality care and efficient use of resources.

VBP models are recent developments in the health system, and they represent a work in progress in terms of our understanding of how best to design these programs to achieve desired goals, the optimal conditions for their successful implementation, and provider response to the incentives. The design features and the context in which a VBP program is implemented are critical determinants of program success.

Given the substantial investments that HHS is making to implement and test a variety of VBP models, this is an opportune moment to reflect on what has been learned from the past decade of experimentation that could guide current and future federal policymaking related

---

[*] Other common terms used for bundled payment arrangements are episode-based payment, episode payment, episode-of-care payment, case rate, evidence-based case rate, global bundled payment, and global payment.

Table 1
2010 Patient Protection and Affordable Care Act Value-Based Purchasing Provisions

Type of VBP Program and Setting	Timeline
Pay for Performance	
Hospital Value-Based Purchasing (HVBP)	October 1, 2012 (current program)
Physicians (or groups of physicians) under Physician Value-Based Payment Modifier	January 1, 2015, for a subset of physicians January 1, 2018, for all physicians (program to be implemented)
Inpatient critical access hospitals	No later than 2 years after date of act (May 1, 2010) (demonstration program)
Hospitals excluded from HVBP program due to insufficient numbers of measures and cases	No later than 2 years after date of act (May 1, 2010) (demonstration program)
Long-term care hospitals	No later than January 1, 2016 (pilot program)
Hospice programs	No later than January 1, 2016 (pilot program)
Psychiatric hospitals	No later than January 1, 2016 (pilot program)
Rehabilitation hospitals	No later than January 1, 2016 (pilot program)
Prospective Payment System–exempt cancer hospitals	No later than January 1, 2016 (pilot program)
Ambulatory surgical centers	Submit plan to Congress no later than January 1, 2011 (plan for program)
Home health agencies	Submit plan to Congress no later than October 1, 2011 (plan for program)
Skilled nursing facilities	Submit plan to Congress no later than October 1, 2011 (plan for program)
Shared Savings	
ACOs	No later than January 1, 2012 (current program)
Bundled Payment	
Hospital/physicians/post-acute care	No later than January 1, 2012 (demonstration program)

to VBP program design and implementation. It is also a good time to consider the type of monitoring and systematic evaluation work that is needed to generate the information that policymakers require to fine tune VBP program designs and to understand the impact these programs are having related to stated goals.

To that end, the Office of the Assistant Secretary for Planning and Evaluation (ASPE) in the HHS asked RAND to review what has been learned about VBP over the past decade. What is the evidence regarding whether these programs have been successful? What are the elements of successful programs? What questions remain unanswered that, if answered, could improve the design and functioning of VBP programs moving forward? This report summarizes the findings from our review. We direct readers to the companion document to this summary report, *Measuring Success in Health Care Value-Based Purchasing Programs: Findings from an Environmental Scan, Literature Review, and Expert Panel Discussions*, for a more detailed description of our analytic methods and findings.

CHAPTER TWO

Study Purpose and Methods

HHS is actively considering the federal government's near- and long-term strategy for how to design and implement VBP programs to achieve the three aims set forth in the National Quality Strategy,[16, 17] which focus on improving the overall quality of care, improving the health of the U.S. population, and making care affordable by reducing the cost of quality health care. In crafting a VBP strategy, HHS seeks to apply the best available evidence to guide policymaking regarding the expansion of VBP across a range of Medicare program settings. To inform VBP policymaking, the federal government is interested in understanding what has been learned from both public- and private-sector P4P programs and their evolution to VBP models and the application of other emerging performance-based payment models, such as ACOs and bundled payment arrangements. Among the questions HHS seeks answers to in order to guide its work are the following:

- **VBP program design:** What do successful VBP programs look like?
  - What is the evidence that VBP programs work to achieve stated goals?
  - What factors (program design features, contextual elements) are associated with successful VBP programs?
  - If VBP programs are not working, what can be done to strengthen programs to be more successful in achieving the desired goals of better value (i.e., improved quality and outcomes, lower cost)?
  - Is there evidence that VBP programs lead to undesired consequences and how could program design mitigate undesired effects?
- **VBP program implementation:** How should VBP programs be implemented to achieve desired results?
  - What elements characterize successful VBP program implementation?
  - How can VBP programs that have been tested in small scale demonstrations and found to have a positive impact be scaled nationally?
  - Can a VBP program designed for one setting (e.g., hospital) be applied in another setting (e.g., ambulatory surgical centers)?
  - Within VBP programs, how can the practices from the highest performing providers be disseminated to garner wide-scale improvements among all providers?
- **Monitoring and evaluation:** What information is needed to understand where VBP works and under what conditions?
  - If VBP programs are not working, what can be done to strengthen them so that they achieve the desired goals of better value?
  - What are the gaps in knowledge and how can they best be addressed?

- How should current and future VBP programs be evaluated to inform future policy decisions?

To address these questions, RAND reviewed the published evidence and consulted with experts on whether VBP programs have been successful in meeting goals, to identify features of successful programs to inform VBP design, and to identify knowledge gaps to inform the focus of future evaluation and monitoring efforts.

Conceptual Framework for Assessing the Effects of Value-Based Purchasing Programs

Because VBP programs are natural experiments and the associated research is observational in nature, Dudley et al.[18] underscore that it is critical that evaluators select theory-driven hypotheses about how incentives affect behavior so as to identify potential confounding factors that could explain observed effects. A framework is a useful construct to help develop theory-driven hypotheses. The panel of technical experts that we convened for this project (see below under "Study Methods") strongly endorsed the need for such a framework.

Several evaluation frameworks have been developed related to VBP programs, including a framework by Dudley et al. focused on assessing P4P experiments,[19] one by McHugh and Joshi that addresses VBP program evaluation,[20] and another by Fisher et al.[21] specifically focused on evaluating ACOs. The three frameworks have similar elements. For example, the Dudley et al. framework describes three core elements—the incentive, predisposing factors, and enabling factors—that influence or mediate the response to provider incentives for quality improvement, while the framework by McHugh and Joshi defines program design, the participants, and contextual factors as elements associated with impacts and implementation. The Fisher ACO evaluation framework similarly considers program components (i.e., ACO contract characteristics, implementation activities), provider characteristics (ACO structure and capabilities), and external factors (i.e., environmental context) that influence intermediate outcomes and impacts. Fisher and colleagues underscore that, because ACOs represent a new model of VBP that is just starting to be tested by both public and private payers, both formative and summative research will be important for guiding policymaking. The McHugh and Joshi framework also emphasizes the importance of implementation (i.e., formative evaluation) research.

Figure 1 represents a general evaluation framework that we adapted from these existing frameworks. For example, in our VBP framework, program design features, characteristics of providers and practice settings, and external factors correspond to the incentive, predisposing and enabling factors described in the Dudley model. Characteristics of providers and practice settings and external factors are important contextual elements that influence the response of providers to the incentives. Our framework attempts to expand on previously developed frameworks by detailing some of the specific factors that should be considered within each of the elements of the framework.

The conceptual framework offers a foundation for considering the design features of the incentive program as well as other factors that influence whether and how providers may respond to the incentives and whether programs are successful in reaching stated goals. The panel of technical experts that we convened for this project identified a set of design features

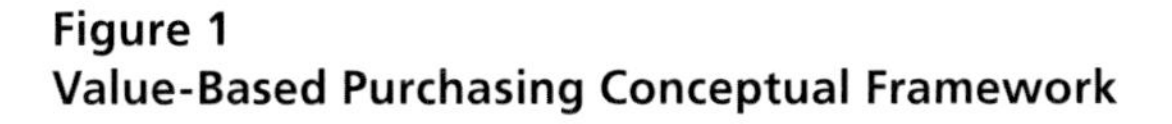

Figure 1
Value-Based Purchasing Conceptual Framework

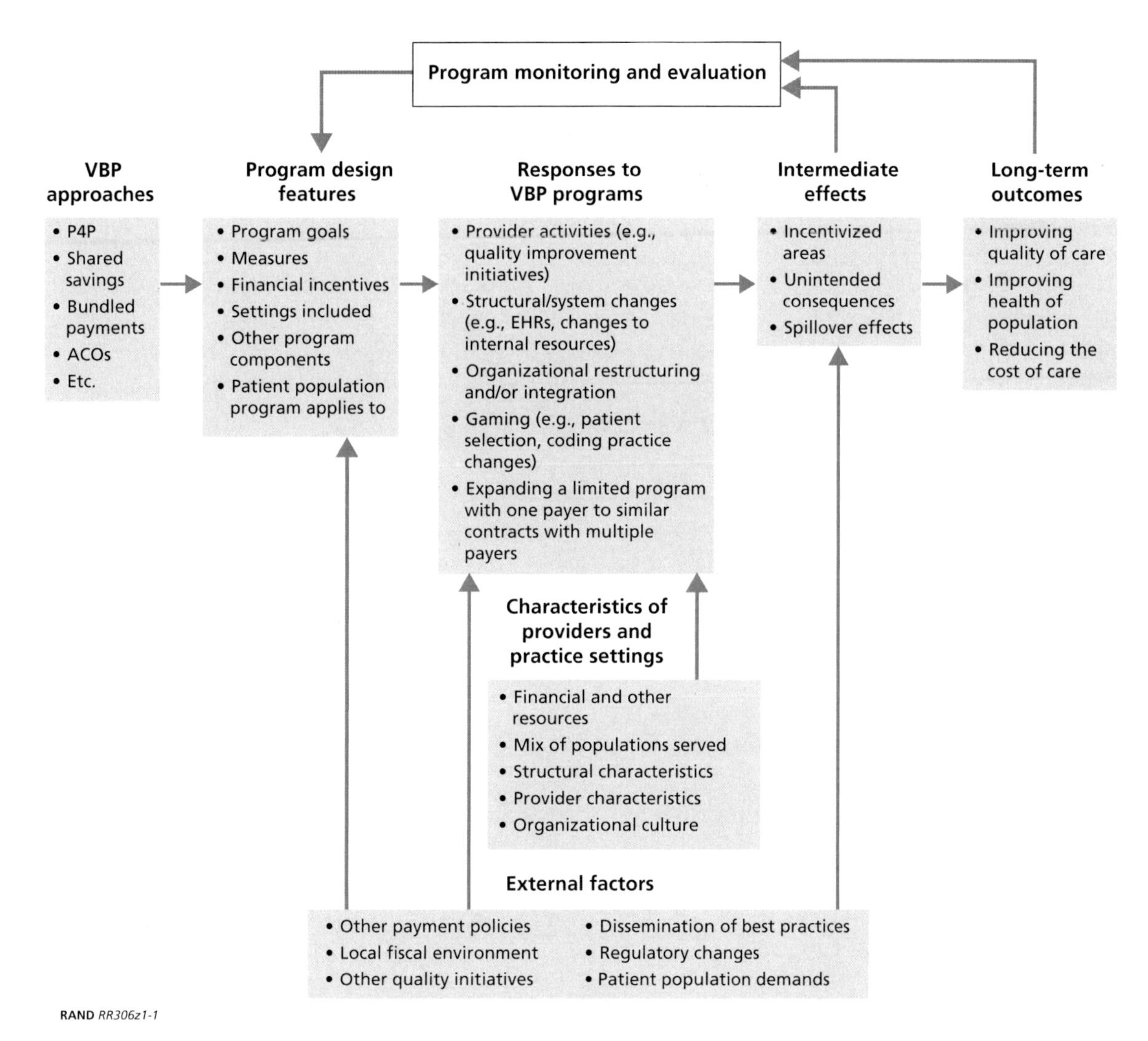

RAND *RR306z1-1*

(i.e., program components) and other factors that they recommended be systematically collected for all VBP programs to facilitate efforts to evaluate VBP programs and to compare and contrast observed impacts across programs (see the appendix). The framework also can be used to guide discussions about the design and implementation of existing VBP programs and those in development and to define a structured agenda for monitoring and evaluating VBP programs, with the explicit goal of developing knowledge to improve the functioning of these programs.

Study Methods

For this study, we defined VBP programs as private or public programs that link financial reimbursement to performance on measures of quality (i.e., structure, process, outcomes, access, and patient experience) and cost or resource use. We focused our review on three broad categories of VBP models: (1) P4P, which includes both "pay for quality" and "pay for quality and resource use, efficiency, or costs"; (2) shared savings models, which typically, but not exclusively, are being deployed in the context of ACOs; and (3) bundled payments for episodes of care (only when paired with holding providers accountable for performance on quality measures). We excluded pay-for-reporting and demand-side programs (e.g., tiered networks and consumer incentives).

ASPE identified a set of research questions for RAND to explore (see companion report, *Measuring Success in Health Care Value-Based Purchasing Programs: Findings from an Environmental Scan, Literature Review, and Expert Panel Discussions*), which were organized around three broad areas of inquiry: (1) measuring the performance of VBP programs, (2) the results of performance in VBP programs, and (3) improving the performance of VBP programs. We used three approaches to gather information to address the questions:

- **Environmental scan of existing VBP programs:** We reviewed information that was publicly available for 129 VBP programs (91 P4P programs, 27 ACOs, and 11 bundled payment programs), of which 85 were sponsored by private health plans, eight by regional collaboratives, and 20 by Medicaid agencies or states. The VBP programs we reviewed do not represent the universe of all VBP programs in current operation in the United States, and the documentation for some programs we reviewed was not complete; therefore, the results should be considered in light of these limitations. Our VBP program review was also limited by the proprietary nature of the information about these programs, which are sponsored by private entities (e.g., health plans).
- **Review of the published evaluation literature on VBP:** We examined the peer-reviewed published literature between January 1, 2000, and April 30, 2013, for studies that evaluated the impact of P4P, ACO, or bundled payment programs, drawing heavily from existing review articles where available. We assessed the methodological quality of each study based on the strength of the evidence it presented, and we graded the strength of the evidence as a whole for each research question. Details are found in the companion document to this report, entitled *Measuring Success in Health Care Value-Based Purchasing Programs: Findings from an Environmental Scan, Literature Review, and Expert Panel Discussions.*
- **Input from the project's technical expert panel (TEP):** We convened an expert panel composed of VBP program sponsors (i.e., private plans and a regional multi-stakeholder collaborative), providers from health systems who have been the target of VBP programs, health services researchers with expertise in examining the effects of VBP programs, and federal participants who represented public payers.

Because many of the design issues and implementation lessons have not found their way into the published literature, the expertise of the VBP program sponsors and providers on the TEP proved to be critical in providing information to address many of the study questions. The TEP met twice in person, in May and June of 2013, for all-day meetings that were facilitated by RAND staff. We provided the expert panelists with the findings from the environmental scan of programs and the literature review as background information for their discussions.[22]

CHAPTER THREE

Summary of Findings

Although the past decade has witnessed a fair amount of experimentation with performance-based payment models, primarily P4P programs, we still know very little about how best to design and implement VBP programs to achieve stated goals and what constitutes a successful program. The published evidence regarding improvements in performance from the P4P experiments of the past decade is mixed; where observed, improvements were typically modest. Many of the published studies evaluating the impact of P4P programs suffer from methodological weaknesses that make it hard to determine whether the VBP intervention had an effect above and beyond other changes (e.g., investment in quality improvement support, public reporting, health information technology [HIT] investments and support) that were simultaneously occurring to improve quality and restrain spending.

VBP programs are natural experiments and inherently difficult to evaluate because program sponsors rarely withhold the VBP intervention from a matched group of providers to see what would have occurred absent the intervention. There are many weaknesses in the methods often used to evaluate P4P (and now the broader class of VBP programs), including reliance on pre-post comparisons without a comparison group that was not exposed to the intervention, comparisons with populations of providers that are substantially different from the treatment group, and failure to account for other factors that may be contributing to the observed results.

ACOs and bundled payment programs that embed clinical quality measures have only recently emerged and are just now being tested and evaluated. There is currently very limited evidence regarding the impact of these programs and whether they can be successfully implemented. Only a handful of ACO evaluation studies have been published, and these evaluations have been of relatively short duration (i.e., 1–2 years), making it difficult to know whether the results are real and can be sustained. These studies also suffer from similar methodological weaknesses as seen in the P4P literature. The published studies show some improvements in cost and quality; however, several of the ACO studies reported cost savings compared with expected year-over-year trends in spending as opposed to comparing the intervention providers' experience against a matched comparison group of providers. Bundled payment programs that incorporate a quality component are equally new, and there is virtually no evidence on whether they can be successfully implemented and what their effects are.

The paucity of publicly available information regarding what constitutes a successful VBP program—that is, what VBP design features and other factors (i.e., characteristics of the providers, the health care market where the VBP program is implemented, and policy/regulatory environment) facilitate success in VBP—presents challenges for policymakers who seek to design VBP programs. In practice, more is likely known about what does and does not work in terms of VBP design and implementation than what the published literature suggests. VBP program sponsors (particularly private program sponsors) have gained a great deal of experience through trial and error as they work to operationalize the VBP concept in real-world settings; however, these experiences are not being documented through traditional means. Because VBP programs are relatively new and experimentation is likely beneficial at this stage of VBP development, the question is how to generate information from all the experimentation. Efforts to extract these lessons from VBP sponsors are critically needed to strengthen the knowledge base.

In the rest of this chapter, we summarize key findings from the environmental scan of existing programs, the literature review, and our discussions with the TEP. The findings are organized by the topic areas we were asked to address in the scope of work for this project. We direct readers of this report to its companion report, *Measuring Success in Health Care Value-Based Purchasing Programs: Findings from an Environmental Scan, Literature Review, and Expert Panel Discussion*, which provides a more detailed summary of the findings from our review and TEP discussions.

Goals of Value-Based Purchasing Programs

Based on our review of VBP programs in operation, VBP program sponsors tend to identify multiple high-level goals that focus on improving clinical quality (75 percent of the programs we reviewed) and cost/affordability (53 percent of the programs we reviewed). Less commonly reported were goals related to improving patient outcomes (34 percent) and patient experience (17 percent). There was some variation in goals among VBP program type, with goals focused on coordination of care and patient experience more prevalent in ACO and bundled payment programs as compared with P4P programs.

In most cases, the goals specified by VBP program sponsors were not quantified or measurable (e.g., "breakthrough improvement in quality" or "bend the cost curve"). In a handful of cases (five of the 129 programs we reviewed), we found quantified goals related to desired cost savings (e.g., "keep 2010 health care premium costs flat" and "reduce the annual increase in cost of care by two percentage points"). Our inability to find the specific performance goals for many of the VBP programs, particularly programs sponsored by private-sector payers, is likely a function of the proprietary nature of this information. Performance measures and thresholds are embedded within the contracts negotiated between providers (i.e., physicians, physician organizations, hospitals) and payers. Because of the absence of quantifiable goals, it is difficult for program sponsors to determine whether programs have been successful in meeting their goals; instead, program sponsors typically examine whether performance on the incentivized measures improved over time. Given this difficulty, the TEP recommended that individual VBP program sponsors establish well-defined, measurable intermediate goals (i.e., program performance targets) derived from external benchmarks and use these to assess success.

Our discussions with the TEP also revealed support for VBP programs having broad goals, and panelists commented that beyond driving improvements in quality and costs, the larger goal of VBP is to transform the way care is delivered to enhance performance. TEP members outlined the following additional goals that they believed would be important to establish and potentially measure to assess VBP program success:

- **Stimulate organizational nimbleness to rapidly learn and improve in order to achieve a new performance target.** TEP members indicated that a key goal of VBP is improving the functional capacity of providers to learn and improve. Therefore, it is important to understand whether there is capacity in health systems and provider organizations to improve quality against a moving target, and whether performance levels can be maintained once targets are achieved. TEP members commented that VBP programs should affect providers' willingness to change, their measurement capacity to identify problems, and their ability to respond to correct quality defects.
- **Promote innovation.** The panelists commented that part of the value of VBP is the innovation that occurs to fix the fundamental problems leading to poor quality and outcomes within provider organizations and, ideally, across providers in response to the incentive scheme. Examples they cited were the creation of more integrated data systems to improve communication between providers, the development of care management protocols that span care settings to improve transitions in care between the hospitals and ambulatory settings, investments in registries that allow physicians to track and better manage high risk populations, the development and use of risk assessment tools, and provision of clinical decision support. There was interest among the TEP panelists in capturing whether and how VBP initiatives are stimulating innovation.

Although the TEP identified a desire to understand whether VBP is successful in helping to make providers "more nimble" and to "improve their functional capacity for learning and improvement," it remains unclear at this stage what providers would need to demonstrate to prove that these aspirational goals had been met. To the extent that these are desired characteristics that VBP program sponsors want to encourage, work is required to define what is meant by these concepts so that VBP sponsors could determine whether this evolution has occurred.

The TEP also discussed whether success should be defined by levels (i.e., absolute performance achieved) or by the counterfactual (i.e., the extent of improvement in performance compared with what it would have been absent the VBP program). A VBP program sponsor may consider a program successful if a certain level of performance is met, whereas researchers would consider a program successful if greater improvements in performance occurred for those providers exposed to VBP as compared with those who were not (i.e., the comparison group). The latter perspective is important because quality may be improving broadly over time as a function of a variety of factors, such as quality improvement interventions and infrastructure improvements distinct from actions undertaken in response to the VBP program, so providers may reach the stated goals in the absence of a VBP program. This discussion highlighted important differences in what program sponsors, policymakers, and researchers are interested in evaluating and what defines success.

The VBP program sponsors on the TEP felt that study designs need to be adapted to fit with the needs for making policy change, such as more rapid but less rigorous initial evaluation cycles to guide decisions about fine-tuning program design. They cited the initial Premier HQID design, which was changed based on less rigorous evidence; the changes were needed to restructure the incentives to achieve more engagement from poorly performing hospitals.

Measures Included in Value-Based Purchasing Programs

Our review of public documents from VBP programs revealed there is a relatively narrow set of measures included in VBP programs that are used as the basis for differential payments. The measures vary somewhat by the health care settings in which they are being deployed as well as by the type of VBP model.* Historically, P4P programs have focused on quality performance, while the newer VBP models (ACOs and bundled payments) incentivize providers for both cost and quality; however, P4P programs have been evolving over time to include more cost and use measures. P4P programs typically include measures of clinical process and intermediate outcomes (e.g., Healthcare Effectiveness Data and Information Set [HEDIS] or Joint Commission measures), patient safety measures (e.g., surgical infection prevention), utilization (generic prescribing, emergency department use, length of stay, ambulatory care sensitive hospital admissions), patient experience (i.e., Consumer Assessment of Healthcare Providers and Systems survey, Hospital Consumer Assessment of Healthcare Providers and Systems survey), and, to a more limited degree, outcomes (e.g., readmissions, mortality, complications, total cost of care or cost per episode) and structural elements (e.g., HIT adoption or meaningful use of HIT requirements for CMS incentive payments, National Committee for Quality Assurance certification or patient-centered medical home certification, staffing, inspections). Clinical measures in the ambulatory setting focus heavily on preventive care and management of heart disease and diabetes, while in the hospital setting, the focus has been on heart attack, congestive heart failure, pneumonia, and surgical infection prevention.

The three ACO program models being tested by CMS use 33 measures, which include HEDIS clinical processes and intermediate outcomes; Consumer Assessment of Healthcare Providers and Systems survey questions on patient experience; all-cause hospital readmission; ambulatory sensitive care hospital admissions; patient safety; and electronic health record (EHR) functionality. Private-sector ACOs are using a similar set of measures, and again the clinical focus has been on three highly prevalent chronic conditions (i.e., heart disease, diabetes, and hypertension), cancer screening, and immunizations. The measures included in bundled payment programs tend to vary by the condition or procedure included in the episode as well as the setting(s) in which care is delivered. Cost measures are most commonly used. In the hospital setting, where most bundled payment programs occur, measures include clinical process, patient safety, readmissions, mortality, length of stay, and total cost of care. Some programs avoid tying physician compensation to outcome measures, so that physicians will not hesitate to treat patients who are more complicated. Little public information is available regarding the measures that are being used in ambulatory care bundled payment programs. Some of the VBP programs we reviewed are signaling that they intend to move to patient-reported outcomes in the next few years, but they are struggling to find market-ready measures that can be readily applied.

The discussions with the TEP highlighted problems with the narrow set of measures typically being used in VBP programs. The TEP estimated that only a small fraction (less than 20 percent) of all care that is delivered by providers is addressed by performance measures in VBP programs. An exception is "total cost of care" contracts (which as of late 2013 apply to only a small number of organizations) that hold providers accountable for the cost of all or

* For example, for fiscal year 2014, CMS has 59 clinical and patient experience measures in its Hospital Inpatient Quality Reporting program and 18 clinical measures for nursing homes under its Nursing Home Quality Initiative.

most care delivered but which only measure quality performance for a fraction of all care delivered by providers. It was the panelists' opinion that the current, narrow set of measures tends to encourage providers to narrowly focus improvement efforts on the things that are measured (teaching to test) rather than wholesale improvement. The TEP also expressed concern that it is hard to demonstrate that VBP programs lead to performance improvements when the incentivized measures are the same set of measures that have been used for nearly a decade (i.e., Joint Commission measures, HEDIS); many of these measures have less room for improvement and, in some cases, have topped out. Panelists commented that shifting measurement focus to areas where performance is lagging[23] would better address the question of whether VBP can improve the delivery of care in areas not previously the focus of reporting and incentives. With respect to what is measured, the TEP questioned whether VBP programs are addressing areas with the greatest impact on health. While medical care can influence health outcomes, the TEP observed that lifestyle behaviors (diet, exercise, smoking, etc.) contribute roughly 50 percent to determining health outcomes.

Another measurement challenge the TEP flagged was the inability to assess value because of the lack of an agreed-upon definition of value and that providers' lack of cost accounting systems that enable them to know the true cost of delivering care. Many organizations have struggled with how best to measure and convey value to providers and consumers, highlighting the need for measure development in this area. Although they did not offer a definition of value, the TEP members thought that a first step would be to achieve consensus on an overarching view of what value means; then VBP sponsors could develop value measures in the context of their own programs.

Many members of the TEP thought that a broad and more comprehensive set of measures in VBP programs would create incentives for providers to perform well across the board, rather than focus narrowly on a small number of areas, which promotes "teaching to the test"—that is, focusing only on improving areas that are measured and incentivized by the VBP program and ignoring clinically important areas that are not. However, neither the literature nor the TEP addressed how many measures are reasonable or practical to implement or when the data collection burden on providers becomes excessive. Expanding the set of measures included in VBP programs to more comprehensively assess care delivered and to include infrequently captured measure domains will require the development of new measures and new types of measures. Developing new measures is a time- and resource-intensive activity. Measurement concepts must be defined, specifications developed, data collection processes piloted, and data validated, among other steps. Recognizing this, the TEP recommended that it would be important to develop a framework to guide future directions about what to measure and, in turn, what measures need to be developed. They stated that the framework should address the multiple levels at which behavioral change needs to occur and where interventions should be directed (i.e., health system, institution, and individual provider).

The TEP identified several areas, discussed below, that should be the focus of future measure expansion work in the context of VBP.

Measuring Patient Outcomes and Functional Status

The TEP members agreed that the ultimate objective of VBP is to hold providers accountable for and financially incentivize provider performance primarily based on measures of health outcomes. CMS expressed that it is moving toward increased accountability for outcomes in its hospital and physician VBP programs, and seeking to find a balance of structure, process, and outcome measures in its programs. An example of this transition to outcomes is illustrated in the hospital VBP program. In the first year of hospital VBP, 70 percent of the measures were process measures, whereas in the second year the percentage drops to 30 percent, as currently outlined in CMS's proposed Notice of Rule Making.[24, 25] Questions remain about the pace at which CMS should push toward outcomes measurement, the types of outcomes to use, and the consequences of those actions.

There was sentiment among the TEP members that functional status/health status is an important, feasible measure and that inclusion of these types of measures would shift VBP programs in the direction of incentivizing performance on outcomes. TEP members pointed to several health care settings and providers that are already measuring functional status on a regular basis: Medicare ACO programs are paid for reporting patient-reported functional limitations, and CMS collects health status information in nursing homes and home health agencies. The Dartmouth Institute is measuring quality-adjusted life years and has built functional status, which is considered a vital sign, into a provider order for life-sustaining care for patients who are at or near the end of life. Other provider representatives stated they are also measuring health status for some conditions. The TEP suggested that CMS could implement the Patient Reported Outcome Measures (PROMs), as the National Health Service in the United Kingdom has done, to measure the performance of hospitals regarding the functioning of patients undergoing selected procedures.

Measuring Appropriateness of Care

TEP members were supportive of including measures of appropriateness (i.e., overuse) in VBP programs, but panelists recognized that additional work is required to develop the definitions and engage providers in using these measures. They cautioned that without an external impetus, providers have little incentive to use practice guidelines or protocols that might withhold care due to the current fee-for-service and malpractice systems, which instead provide an incentive to increase the use of diagnostics and procedures. The TEP commented that providers under risk-sharing arrangements (e.g., ACO and total cost of care contracts) will be more likely to implement appropriateness guidelines, because the financial incentives they face are aligned with focusing on reducing the overuse of services that are not deemed appropriate. Based on direct experience, members of the TEP observed that when implementing appropriateness criteria measures in a health system, it can take years to get providers to buy-in related to establishing the criteria and being held accountable for performance against the criteria. TEP members suggested that measurement of shared decisionmaking is one of the keys to implementing appropriateness of care. A TEP representative of one health system noted the provider is piloting a process of "patient appropriate order entry" where the specialist has to attest that he or she held a discussion with the patient about the appropriateness of the care being recommended. Another TEP member recognized the challenge that physicians could face if appropriateness of care metrics are in conflict with patient preferences.

Enhancing the Ability of Electronic Health Records to Support Performance Measurement and Improvement

There was widespread agreement among the TEP members that it is important to incentivize and help providers build the infrastructure for quality improvement. EHRs may facilitate measurement and improvement, but the TEP did not see this happening in the near term. Based on their experiences to date, the panelists expressed concern that most EHRs are far from including a comprehensive set of standardized data in data fields that can readily produce data needed to support the construction of performance measures, in part because providers who are the customers for EHRs are not demanding that EHRs be able to generate this type of information. Meaningful use requirements* currently require that EHR vendors build functionalities in EHRs to support reporting from a select list of quality measures. This is very different than freeing up the EHR data for use by providers for their own performance monitoring, improvement, and broader performance measurement. For example, some delivery systems have EHRs and registries that give providers alerts at the point of care on the patients' status with respect to a given measure and/or that allow providers to benchmark their performance on measures against their peers. ASPE staff commented that ASPE is working with the Office of the National Coordination for Health Information Technology, which is the lead federal agency responsible for meaningful use requirements, to make EHRs function more effectively to facilitate automated capture and reporting of quality measures, but this will be a long process.

Types of Incentives

The review of public documents from program sponsors found that the types of financial incentives offered to providers have expanded beyond bonuses that have been commonly used in P4P programs, and which work at the margin, to a stronger set of incentives that more fundamentally alter payment arrangements. Examples include changes to fee schedules, shared savings arrangements (either alone or combined with bonuses or shared risk, in which the ACO loses money if targets for reducing patient costs are not met), and global budgets (i.e., overarching payment for all care delivered to a patient, similar to capitation). Most of the ACOs reviewed in our environmental scan have shared savings arrangements, and a few have shared risk. VBP programs often use combinations of financial incentives to drive change. The Blue Cross Blue Shield of Massachusetts Alternative Quality Contract (AQC)—an ACO-type arrangement—allows for shared savings and shared risk and offers a bonus payment up to 10 percent above the global budget based on performance on quality measures. The majority of the bundled payment programs for which we were able to identify information are offering shared savings to providers, while others adjust the episode fee based on quality performance.

Although our review of the literature on VBP did not include a review of the use of consumer incentives, the TEP highlighted the importance of working to align incentives for consumers. Panelists commented that creating incentives to drive patients toward higher-performing providers could strengthen the impetus for providers to improve and might be more effective in shifting performance up than current P4P incentives that attempt to influence provider performance at the margin. CMS commented that it is already taking a number of actions in its VBP programs to affect consumer market behavior. For example, if a Medicare Advantage plan is consistently low-performing for three years, beneficiaries are not allowed to

---

* The Medicare and Medicaid EHR Incentive Programs provide incentive payments to eligible professionals, eligible hospitals, and critical access hospitals as they adopt, implement, upgrade, or demonstrate meaningful use of certified EHR technology. Eligible professionals can receive up to $44,000 through the Medicare EHR Incentive Program and up to $63,750 through the Medicaid EHR Incentive Program. (CMS, "Medicare and Medicaid EHR Incentive Program Basics," web page, no date. As of November 15, 2013: http://www.cms.gov/Regulations-and-Guidance/Legislation/EHRIncentivePrograms/Basics.html.)

enroll online in that plan. Additionally, CMS sends letters to beneficiaries who are enrolled in low-performing Medicare Advantage plans and encourages them to shift to high-performing "five Star" plans; to facilitate plan switching, beneficiaries in low-performing contracts have the option of changing plans any time during the year. Panelists recommended that CMS continue to explore using tools like these to push quality improvement in a strategic way.

Type of Benchmarks/Thresholds

An important design element of any VBP program is the performance benchmarks or thresholds that are used to determine who will receive an incentive payment. In some cases, these are absolute, fixed benchmarks (e.g., provider must have at least 90 percent performance on mammography screening), while in other cases benchmarks are relative (e.g., the provider's performance must in in the top 20th percentile of performance), and as a result the absolute score required to reach the percentile cut point changes year to year. Some VBP programs reward providers for attaining specific benchmarks, improving over time, or a combination of attainment and improvement.

We were only able to find information about the types of benchmarks used for a third of the VBP programs in our environmental scan. There was no publicly available information about the benchmarks being used by bundled payment programs. Among P4P programs, the most common benchmark used was an absolute threshold only, followed by relative thresholds only, which may be based on the performance of peers in the market, the state, or nationally. Other programs, such as the CMS Hospital VBP program, have two paths to earning incentives: attainment against an absolute threshold or showing improvement over time.

Very little information was publicly available about the types of benchmarks being used for ACO models, as these are developed in the context of private negotiations between payers and providers. The exception was the three CMS ACO demonstration models. In its shared savings programs, CMS is establishing the cost benchmark for each agreement period for each ACO using three-years-prior expenditure data. Quality benchmarks are based on national percentile rankings from the year prior, and points are assigned on a sliding scale based on the ACO's performance. For 2013, the Pioneer ACO program measures and rewards improvement on the quality measures. The Physician Group Practice demonstration, the precursor ACO demonstration that CMS ran, utilized absolute thresholds for quality measures.

The literature highlights some of the issues associated with use of different types of benchmarks. Providers report disliking relative thresholds,[1, 3] for several reasons. First, providers do not know ahead of time what actual level of performance is required to obtain the incentive payment, creating much uncertainty about whether their performance is "good enough." Second, when topped-out measures are included in the VBP program, providers may have very high performance that does not meet the necessary threshold to receive the incentive, but yet is not meaningfully different from the performance of providers that do receive the incentive payment. For example, the initial design of the Premier HQID in Phase 1 of the program's implementation only paid hospitals that were in the top 20th percentile of performance. Performance rates for a large proportion of the hospitals hovered around 99 percent on a number of the measures, and which hospitals received the incentive payment was based on differences in performance at the second decimal point. In response to this problem, CMS changed the incentive structure in Phase 2 of the Premier HQID to reward above-average achievement and improvement.

A relative incentive structure can promote a "race to the top," creating perverse incentives for providers to allocate resources to improvement on a measure that may not yield the greatest clinical benefit and which may lead to overtreatment of patients. Achieving 100 percent performance on a measure also may not be appropriate and may lead to overtreatment. No matter how well the performance measure is constructed, and despite attempts to exclude from the denominator patients who should be excluded, it is unlikely that any process measure will be applicable to 100 percent of the population. In practice, there are often sound reasons why some small percentage of patients does not receive recommended processes of care. These reasons include patient preferences regarding treatment, contraindications to recommended therapy (e.g., allergies or intolerance of medications), prior rare side effects, and the clinical challenges of balancing treatment of multiple clinical conditions and interactions between medications. Typically, the patients in the upper tail of the distribution differ from patients in the other 95 percent of the distribution in ways that performance measurement typically is not very good at systematically capturing through exclusion criteria. In these cases, not providing the recommended care is not an error in care. In the UK Quality Outcomes Framework P4P program, where providers are allowed to exclude patients from the measure calculation (i.e., exception reporting), a median of 5.3 percent of patients were excluded from performance measure calculations. Exception reporting occurred most often for performance measures related to providing treatments and achieving target levels of intermediate outcomes.[27] U.S.-based VBP programs do not typically allow providers to exclude patients from reporting.

TEP members noted that while establishing absolute attainment thresholds is preferred by providers, some payers express concern that this approach removes the motivation for providers to continue to improve once the threshold has been attained. Paying all who achieve an absolute attainment target also creates budgeting challenges for payers, who will not be able to estimate how many providers they will need to pay; if the payer sets a fixed incentive pool, the more providers who succeed results in a smaller incentive payment per provider. Some VBP sponsors have set multiple absolute targets along a continuum to motivate improvement at all levels of performance and to continue to motivate improvement at the top end of the performance distribution.

Performance of Value-Based Purchasing Programs

VBP program sponsors and evaluators have primarily assessed whether improvements have occurred in the measures that were incentivized through VBP. Efforts to disentangle the VBP effect from other interventions designed to improve the delivery of health care locally and nationally (e.g., investments in HIT, enhanced quality improvement, and public reporting) have proven more challenging to study, because the natural experiments typically lack robust comparison groups. Furthermore, contextual factors and how they may contribute to any observed impacts are rarely considered.

The TEP highlighted some of the challenges with evaluations conducted over the past decade: (1) the measures included in a VBP program are often also included in national performance measurement and public reporting programs (e.g., CMS) and the VBP programs by other private sponsors, making it difficult to tease out the effect of any individual VBP program; (2) the presence of other incentives (e.g., public reporting/transparency of performance results) make it difficult to isolate the effects on incentivized measures of the financial incentives; (3) there is usually no comparison population when a VBP program is implemented statewide or nationally; (4) the size of payment incentives is often small; (5) VBP programs typically have used the same core measures (i.e., HEDIS, Joint Commission measures) that have been used for more than a decade and are largely "topped out"; and (6) there is a substantial lag for the data required to assess impact, such as data on avoiding admissions and readmissions.

Clinical Quality

Pay-for-Performance

We identified 49 studies that examined the effect of P4P on process and intermediate outcome measures: 37 studies examined the effect of P4P on process measures for physicians or physician groups;[2, 6, 9, 11, 28–57] 11 studies examined the effect of P4P on process measures in the hospital setting;[58–65] and a single study examined the effect of P4P on process measures in other care settings.[66] The published studies have focused on assessing a few large P4P interventions (e.g., the Premier demonstration, the Physician Group Practice demonstration, the Integrated Healthcare Association P4P program, the Blue Cross Hawaii P4P program, the Massachusetts multi-plan P4P program, the UK Quality Outcomes Framework P4P program, and more recently the Blue Cross Blue Shield of Massachusetts AQC) and a number of very small-scale incentive experiments that were of short duration.

Overall, the results of the studies were mixed, and studies with stronger methodological designs were less likely to identify significant improvements associated with the P4P programs. Any identified effects were relatively small. Studies with weaker study designs mostly found that P4P was significantly associated with higher levels of quality, and many reported substantial effect sizes.

Accountable Care Organizations

We identified six evaluations (of five distinct ACO programs) examining the effect on quality of care associated with implementing an ACO or ACO-like model (e.g., the Blue Cross Blue Shield of Massachusetts AQC, which is a global budget total cost of care contract, and the CMS Physician Group Practice demonstration, which was a precursor to the CMS ACO demonstrations). Five of the studies investigated the effect of the ACO on a small number of process-of-care measures[67–71] and showed greater improvements than controls on some but not all of the measures. In addition to these evaluations, CMS issued a press release on the early experiences of the Medicare Pioneer ACO on July 16, 2013.[72] In the first performance year, the Pioneer ACOs had higher performance overall than the Medicare fee-for-service beneficiary comparison population on the 15 quality of care measures reported, but it was not reported whether the Pioneer ACOs had greater improvements or just higher baseline performance. At this stage, it is difficult to discern the effects of ACOs on quality, given the newness of the ACO model and the short period of implementation.

Bundled Payments

Of the three studies of bundled payments that include value-based payment design elements (cost and quality components), only one study examined the effect of bundled payments on process measures. The study found that adherence on 40 clinical process measures increased from 59 percent to 100 percent.[73] However, this study was conducted in a single integrated health system with unique characteristics that make generalizing the findings to other providers difficult. A recent systematic review of the bundled payment literature showed inconsistent effects on quality measures associated with implementing bundled payment arrangements. Most of the bundled payment programs reviewed in this study did not include quality elements as part of the incentive formula; in these instances, the evaluators sought to determine whether the application of bundled payments resulted in undesired effects on quality.[13]

Outcomes

We reviewed 21 studies that evaluated the effect of P4P on outcomes in physician groups (12), hospitals (6), and other settings (3). In the physician practice setting, the studies generally focused on a small number of intermediate diabetes outcomes and found mixed results. Of the studies we rated as fair- and poor-quality in terms of their design, three[35, 39, 52] found between 2 and 22 percent improvement in the percentage of patients with glycated hemoglobin (HbA1c) control, while another study found no effect.[33] There was only a single study rated as good-quality,[74] and it found that changes in diabetes intermediate outcome measures (e.g., percentage of patients with HbA1c and lipid control) were not statistically significant from the comparison group. Four studies focused on other types of health outcome measures. One good-quality study[75] found that a P4P program focused on prenatal care for pregnant members of a union health plan led to a reduction in admissions to the neonatal intensive care unit (NICU), but no reduction in low birth weight. Three fair- and poor-quality studies[30, 45, 56] found no effect on mortality, readmission, or incident of major health events (e.g., stroke or heart attack), but did find a slight reduction in initial hospitalizations.

The studies in the hospital setting focused primarily on measuring the effects on mortality. Three of the studies that focused on outcomes were deemed to be of good methodological quality and found mixed results. Glickman[58] found no evidence that in-hospital mortality improvements were incrementally greater at P4P hospitals in the CMS Premier HQID program, while Ryan[76] found no evidence that the HQID had a significant effect on risk adjusted 30-day mortality acute myocardial infarction, heart failure, pneumonia, or coronary artery bypass graft (CABG). Sutton et al.[77] found that risk-adjusted mortality for the conditions included in the P4P program decreased by 1.3 percent compared with controls in a study evaluating a program in the UK modeled after CMS HQID. Another study by Jha et al.,[78] which we deemed to be of fair quality, found no differences in a composite measure of 30-day mortality between hospitals in the HQID demonstration and hospitals exposed to pay-for-reporting. Mortality declined similarly across the two groups of hospitals (0.04 percent per quarter), and mortality rates were similar after six years of the pay-for-reporting demonstration. When considering the results from this study, it is important to note that hospitals exposed to the pay-for-reporting incentive increased their performance on the process measures similarly to pay-for-reporting hospitals, and both sets of hospitals topped out performance on these measures, so that there was no variation in performance to detect a differential effect.

One study,[79] which we rated as good, evaluated five states' Medicaid P4P programs in nursing homes and found that three of six outcome measures (the percentage of residents being physically restrained, in moderate to severe pain, and having developed pressure sores) improved a modest amount, between 0.3 and 0.5 percent one year after P4P implementation. Performance on other targeted quality measures either did not change or worsened. Based on this study, it is unclear what the effects of P4P in the nursing home setting are. We also reviewed two studies that we deemed to be of fair quality. Hittle et al.[80] found that only two measures (improvement in pain interfering with activity and improvement in urinary incontinence), which were non-incentivized, showed significant differences between treatment and control home health agencies across one intervention year; otherwise, no differences were found in the incentivized measures. Shen[81] found that P4P was associated with a reduction in the proportion of clients in substance abuse clinics classified as most severely ill for three years post-intervention.

Among the studies evaluating ACOs, there is limited evidence that ACOs may reduce hospital readmission rates.[67, 68] Only one bundled payment study investigated the effect on health outcomes, and it found no effect.[73]

Costs

Pay-for-Performance

Few studies have investigated the impact of P4P on costs. The studies with the strongest study designs report mixed effects on costs in the physician or physician group setting.[46, 75] Two studies with weak designs[4, 45] found evidence of significant cost savings and a positive return on investment. We found only two studies that specifically investigated changes in costs in the hospital setting. Both of these studies were based on the HQID, and neither found any significant effects on hospital costs, revenues, margins or Medicare payments.[82, 83]

Accountable Care Organizations

All of the studies we reviewed attribute various degrees of cost savings for the shared savings payment model, but not all of the individual ACOs were able to generate statistically significant savings relative to controls. [67–69, 70, 71] CMS also reported that the costs for the Pioneer ACO beneficiaries increased 0.3 percent in 2012 compared with 0.8 percent growth for similar Medicare fee-for-service beneficiaries. While 13 of the 32 ACOs shared savings with CMS, two Pioneer ACOs had shared losses. Two Pioneer ACOs were leaving the ACO program, and an additional seven were switching to the Medicare Shared Savings Program, which involved less risk to providers. Because there were only six studies of four programs, the studies were of short duration, and several had poor or no comparison group, the evidence is insufficient to make conclusions about the impact of ACO payment structures on costs.

Bundled Payments

Of the two studies investigating the impact of bundled payments, both identified reductions in costs. One found a reduction in hospital charges of around five percent,[73] while the other found a reduction in costs per case of roughly $2,000 over a two-year period.[84] The systematic review that documented the impact of implementation of 19 bundled payment programs[13] found that all programs showed declines of 10 percent or less in spending and utilization.

Unintended Effects

We examined undesired behaviors (often referred to as unintended consequences) and spillover effects to assess any unintended effects from these programs. Undesired effects include provider gaming of the data used to generate scores, ignoring other clinically important areas that are not measured and incentivized by the P4P program, avoiding sicker or more challenging patients when providing care, providing care that is not clinically recommended, and overtreating patients. Other undesired effects are an increase in disparities in treatment or outcomes among patients and the VBP program having harmful effects on providers who serve more challenging patient populations. Spillover effects occur when changes made to improve areas measured by VBP programs extend to other areas not included in the VBP program. The literature was sparse related to undesired and spillover effects; few studies have looked at the main effects of VBP interventions, let alone their side effects.

Pay-for-Performance

We identified 21 articles that examined undesired behaviors and spillover effects in P4P programs. Most of the published evidence regarding undesired effects related to application of P4P shows either small or no effects. However, recent studies in the Veteran's Administration found evidence of overtreatment of patients with hypertension and diabetes associated with use of intermediate outcome measures that use thresholds.[85–87] These authors have called for moving from the current class of dichotomous target measures (i.e., met or didn't meet a threshold such as HbA1c <7), where there is a push to get all patients to the threshold, to a set of improved performance measures that focus on giving providers credit for appropriate clinical actions taken (intensification of medications, being on maximal medications, contraindications to further treatment, etc.) and which account for individual risks and preferences. An improved set of performance measures could help reduce incentives to overtreat patients. In addition to the selection of appropriate performance measures, VBP program sponsors should conduct monitoring studies[88] to assess whether and how often patients may be receiving inappropriate treatment so that they can adjust the measures included in VBP programs to mitigate these effects. The lack of evidence on observed negative effects in other P4P studies may be due to the fact that many of the P4P interventions studied were small in scale, of short duration, and did not have substantial amounts of revenue at risk that might encourage providers to engage in undesired behaviors.

Our review of the literature found a small number of studies (n=5) that examine whether P4P programs have spillover effects. The P4P studies have found mixed effects, with some finding no effects (either positive or negative) on measures that were non-incentivized,[58, 89] one finding negative effects,[90] and, in a few cases, evidence of improvement on non-incentivized measures within the same conditions that were the target of the incentives.[48, 91] The evaluation of the UK Quality Outcomes Framework P4P program found that that both incentivized and non-incentivized measures improved between 2004 and 2005 for asthma, diabetes, and heart disease, but that the mean quality scores for aspects of care that were not linked to incentives (only for asthma and heart disease) declined between 2005 and 2007 while the mean scores for the incentivized measures continued to increase. Group practices participating in the CMS Physician Group Practice demonstration reported implementing a variety of quality improvement and care management programs, information technology, and patient registries, all of which have the potential to improve quality of care beyond the measures included in the demonstration; however, no spillover effects were measured.

Accountable Care Organizations

Because these models are newly being implemented and have yet to gain experience, there are no studies that have examined unintended consequences in ACO models, and only one study that assessed spillover effects. A recent study by McWilliams et al.[92] found spillover effects to the Medicare population from implementation of the Blue Cross Blue Shield of Massachusetts's AQC, which targeted commercial HMO enrollees. This study examined changes associated with the AQC in spending and quality of care for traditional fee-for-service Medicare beneficiaries and found that the AQC was associated with lower spending for Medicare beneficiaries but not with consistently improved quality. The AQC evaluation research team also has examined the effect on quality measures not included in AQC, particularly for children with special needs; in this case, they observed more improvement for generic prescribing measures, but no effect on other measures that were not incentivized. Within the AQC practices, improvements were larger for AQC members (HMO members), and there did not seem to be spillover effects to the Blue Cross Blue Shield of Massachusetts PPO members; by extension, the study team doubted there would be spillover improvements for PPO patients for other health plans. A TEP member who represented the AQC cited two possible reasons for the absence of spillover effects: (1) Blue Cross Blue Shield of Massachusetts has provided physician practices with better data on AQC members than other plans' members, so a provider's behavior changes only for the AQC patients, since they have better data to manage those patients; and (2) the practices have used case managers and other resources for high-risk subgroups covered by the AQC, and these resources are not available for other high-risk patient populations they serve. Other TEP members agreed that this is a common occurrence, as health plans focus on providing resources for their members who are the focus of the VBP programs.

ACOs are expected to implement a variety of quality improvement and care management programs, information technology, and patient registries, which have the potential to improve quality of care more broadly and which could generate positive spillover effects. Some researchers and policymakers have expressed concerns that the formation of ACOs may lead to greater market concentration and have the adverse effect of raising prices; the TEP expressed similar concerns. One TEP member commented that in Massachusetts, a law was passed in 2012 that sets a maximum rate of growth in health care spending by providers and hospitals, which holds providers accountable. This law established guardrails and protects against the effects of excessive consolidation. The TEP suggested that a similar law in other states or nationally could be a strong policy lever to guard against this type of behavior.

Bundled Payments

We found no evidence of unintended effects or spillover effects from the three studies of bundled payments that included quality measures. The Hussey et al.[13] review of the broader bundled payment literature highlighted the types of undesired effects that it has been hypothesized might occur in the context of bundled payment arrangements: increasing the number of bundles (volume), underuse of appropriate care services that may lead to poorer outcomes for patients, selection of low-risk patients into the bundles and avoidance of high-risk (potentially more expensive) patients, upcoding to maximize payment for the bundle, and moving services in time or location to qualify for separate reimbursement. However, Hussey et al. found limited evidence on unbundling services and upcoding, but consistent evidence regarding shifting services to other settings of care (e.g., from inpatient to outpatient). There was little evidence that there were major effects on quality; rather, the findings were mixed, with some measures having improved while other worsened.

The TEP supported the need to monitor spillover effects in VBP programs. To assess spillover effects on quality requires access to data for other measures (within the same clinical condition or addressing other clinical conditions) that were not incentivized by the program, something that most programs do not routinely collect. The TEP also identified multiple possible unintended consequences, the occurrence of which should be monitored, including the loss of revenue for providers caring for disadvantaged populations, the excessive exclusion of patients when that is an option in the program, access barriers and patient turnover from practices related to providers avoiding more difficult patients, and market concentration and price effects in the context of ACOs.

Effect on Disparities

Many P4P studies have commented about possible unintended effects for patients of low socioeconomic status (SES) and the providers that serve these populations (e.g., safety net clinics and hospitals). Examinations of whether VBP programs work to reduce or increase disparities are challenged by the lack of information at the patient level on race, ethnicity, education, SES, and other markers of vulnerable populations prone to disparities.

We found only five empirical studies that assessed the effects of P4P on disparities. Among the four studies that evaluated U.S. P4P programs, three found no effects related to increasing or decreasing racial/ethnic or SES disparities while one[93] poor-quality study found very small significant differences in baseline performance for hospitals with a high disproportionate share hospital (DSH) index comparing HQID P4P and pay-for-reporting hospitals (between –0.5 percent and –1.1 percent lower performance for high DSH-index hospitals versus non-high-DSH-index hospitals).* Three years post-HQID-intervention based solely on attaining performance in the top 20th percentile of performance distribution, there were modestly greater gains (only a few significant) for the high-DSH-index hospitals compared with the non-high-DSH-index hospitals exposed to P4P (e.g., 0.6 percent to 1.2 percent higher), and no differences in performance were observed between high-DSH-index and non-high-DSH-index hospitals exposed to P4P. This study should be interpreted in light of the fact that differences at baseline were negligible, and nearly all hospitals in both the P4P and pay-for-reporting groups topped out their performance on the clinical process measures that were the focus of this study.

The 2010 Ryan study,[94] which had a strong design, found no negative access effects related to avoiding treating minority patients after introduction of the Premier HQID. A more recent (2012) study by Ryan et al.[63] found that changes to the HQID incentive structure between Phase I and II of the program resulted in a redistribution of available incentive payments, with a greater proportion going to hospitals with greater socioeconomic disadvantage (as measured by the DSH index). This effect was a function of changes in the structure of the incentive and not due to lower-performing hospitals actually improving more.[95] This study found that disparities neither had worsened nor reduced. A study from the United Kingdom[96] showed a lessening of the disparities gap in performance among primary care practices, with measures largely topping out on performance; however, the results of this study are not generalizable to the United States due to substantial differences in the delivery system (national health system, national HIT platform in primary care practices) and design of the P4P program. There are currently no empirical studies on disparities for either ACO or bundled payment VBP models.

---

* DSH hospitals are those that receive compensation through Medicare for treating a disproportionate number of indigent patients.

A TEP member from one large commercial health plan noted that a global-budget contract model with strong quality incentives had driven important gains in closing racial and ethnic disparities. This is because a few medical groups with a low-SES patient mix worked to innovate with their population and to get their doctors to improve quality. These provider groups with low-SES patient populations actually achieved some of the highest gains and absolute quality scores in the state. However, this was not a universal finding among all groups with low-SES patients.

While the TEP recognized the importance of monitoring the effects of VBP programs on disparities in care, panelists also noted that assessing the effect of VBP on disparities is difficult to monitor due to the lack of routinely collected data on the demographic and socioeconomic characteristics of patients. TEP members indicated that they had faced challenges in capturing this information, despite their interest in capturing self-reported language, health literacy, and indicators of patient vulnerability to help improve their ability to work with patients. However, several providers on the TEP stated they were making inroads in the data they capture to be able to examine disparities. For example, one delivery system has a mandatory data gathering protocol for zip code, race, and ethnicity.

Characteristics of High- and Low-Performing Providers

There is limited evidence characterizing high- and low-performing providers under VBP. The few studies that do describe characteristics of high- and low-performing providers have been opportunistic in defining the characteristics based on the variables that were available to them (e.g., provider size and type), rather than considering a broad set of factors that might differentiate high and low performers. The TEP noted that the American Medical Group Association has developed a set of elements for what defines the characteristics of a high-performing health system;[97] however, it remains untested whether these elements differentiate high and low performers under VBP.

Most of the studies that looked at provider characteristics focused on physician or physician group P4P programs. The limited literature shows that higher-performing providers tend to be large provider organizations,[8, 49, 74] have a medical group rather than an Independent Practice Association (IPA) organizational structure, have more HIT infrastructure,[98–101] and have been historically high performers. Other studies find that high performers engage in more care management processes,[8] use order sets and clinical pathways for measured areas,[102] have nursing staff's support for quality indicators, have adequate human resources for initiatives to improve performance,[102] and engage in more external quality improvement initiatives.[8] High performers also served a smaller fraction of low-SES or Medicaid patients.[49, 93] Lower-performing providers under P4P programs tended to serve a lower-SES population (i.e., physician organizations with more Medicaid patients[49, 74, 103] or hospitals with a high DSH index[93]). Hospitals that achieved the largest improvements under P4P are characterized as being well financed, operating in less competitive markets,[61] having lower performance at baseline,[63, 64] and having a higher DSH index.[93]

Although associations have been found between patient population SES and provider performance, it is important to note that some providers that serve low-SES populations are able to perform well. For example, Medicare has found that most hospitals with high proportions of Medicaid patients achieve readmission rates comparable to those with fewer Medicaid patients.[103]

The CMS Physician Group Practice demonstration evaluation highlighted organizational characteristics associated with performance. Physician groups characterized as being either affiliated with an academic medical center or a freestanding physician group practice were more able to achieve both quality and cost targets than groups with only non-academic hospital affiliations. It is unclear whether the results based on the ten physician groups that self-selected into the Physician Group Practice demonstration would generalize more broadly. Case studies and commentaries suggest that strong physician leadership with a clear strategy and vision is necessary to change practice culture to one that is comfortable with sharing the risk of a predetermined patient population.[104–107] There have been no studies of VBP-type bundled payment models conducted that compare the features of high and low performers under these programs; implementation of these models has proven challenging, and there are few models that have been evaluated.

Features of Successful Value-Based Purchasing Programs

There is very limited published literature to inform what structural and implementation features are associated with successful P4P programs. It is rare to find studies that examine the effects of alternative design features (e.g., the size or frequency of the incentive payment) to assess their impact on provider behavior; the studies that exist are typically small-scale, of short duration,[108] and in many cases the intervention being tested was not expected to be permanent, so providers would not have been expected to invest in practice redesign to improve outcomes and obtain rewards. Consequently, it is difficult to assess from these studies whether the programs have been successful and would be if scaled up to a larger number of providers (i.e., statewide or nationally), what would have happened if the intervention was sustained, and what can be generalized to implementing P4P in the same setting or other settings.

Based on the review of the published literature, there have been mixed findings on the effectiveness of VBP programs to meet its intended goals to improve quality and control costs. This may be because VBP programs are still a work in progress and sponsors are continuing to evolve these programs in response to what does and does not work when implemented. Despite the fact that many programs have been in operation for the past five to ten years, there is a substantial gap in the knowledge base about what has been learned regarding design and implementation in large P4P programs to inform what features promote success in VBP programs.

ACOs are new, and there has not been sufficient time to test ACOs to know whether they can succeed and what factors must be present to allow them to form and achieve desired goals. There is, as yet, little accumulated knowledge about their formation and, once formed, what types of performance results are accrued and what factors are associated with observed performance results. Evaluations of the private- and public-sector ACO experiments will hopefully generate knowledge to inform what factors need to be present for an ACO to succeed in meeting performance goals. Various challenges associated with implementing bundled payments have been identified,[14] and, similar to ACOs, these models are not well tested or in routine operation.

When we queried the TEP about the features of successful VBP programs based on their knowledge from having designed and operated these programs, most panelists agreed that the evidence is thin regarding successful programs and what features characterize these programs. Based on the panelists' anecdotal evidence and the limited literature, we identified six features that appear to influence the success of VBP programs:

- **Sizable incentives:** A limited number of studies have shown that larger incentives were associated with a larger impact on performance.[48, 61] Incentives that were large enough to compensate providers for the effort required to obtain them was identified as one characteristic associated with more successful programs in a study of P4P in five Medicaid plans.[50] Researchers who have found limited effects associated with P4P programs have hypothesized that incentives were too small to garner the attention of providers, but there is uncertainty about how big incentives need to be to garner the desired response and investment for improvement by providers while also minimizing the likelihood of unintended consequences. Absolute incentive size is influenced by the size of the program's incentives (e.g., 1 or 2 percent of base payment), the size of the base payment (e.g., diagnostic related group [DRG] payment amount), and the number of a provider's patients who are covered by the program, as incentives are often computed on a per capita basis. An important policy consideration regarding the size of the incentive relates to the fact that in U.S. VBP programs, payers fund the incentive payment in a budget-neutral fashion, meaning that the winnings of high-quality providers are financed by the loss of revenue from poor-quality providers. In this situation, increasing the size of the incentives could potentially lead to large redistributions of resources among providers and have the undesired effect of de-resourcing low-quality providers who may be most in need of resources to be able to improve quality.
- **Measure alignment:** A number of TEP members discussed the importance of measure alignment across VBP programs to give providers a clear signal of what is important. However, if different VBP programs cover different patient populations, then it is more important for measures to align with the population's conditions than with other VBP programs. If programs are measuring an area where established measures exist, they should use the measures as defined and not tweak the measures to promote alignment.
- **Provider engagement:** A few studies have identified the involvement of key stakeholders in the P4P system design and implementation as important.[5, 109] Similarly, a number of TEP members discussed the importance of provider engagement in design and implementation of VBP (e.g., providing input on the design of the program, participating in choosing performance measures and targets).
- **Performance targets:** TEP members discussed the importance of the methodology used to measure and reward performance. Members stressed the importance of rewarding both achievement and improvement (such as was used in the second phase of the Premier HQID) and that VBP programs should not be designed as a "tournament" wherein relative thresholds are used and providers are pitted against each other (which was how the incentive was structured in Phase 1 of the HQID and in many other P4P programs). Some TEP members recommended that the reward should be based on objective targets that are defined prior to the start of the measurement year in absolute terms; if a provider hits those targets, it should receive an incentive payment. Providers can then strive to achieve a number of targets along a continuum and compete against themselves rather than competing with other providers for a limited number of "winning positions" (e.g.,

top 20th percentile of performance). This approach provides motivation for all providers to move up the scale.

- **Data and other quality improvement support:** There was an extensive discussion among the TEP of the importance of support to help providers improve, particularly through the use of HIT and data registries. It was also noted that best practices for sharing, consultative support, health coaching, and other infrastructure building are important types of support to make available to providers participating in VBP.

Dissemination of Best Practices from Highest-Performing Providers

TEP members stated that the dissemination of best practices currently occurs through trade conferences and regional quality improvement activities. Although the information from these conferences is not published, several provider organization TEP members observed that they do provide vital information for organizational learning of best practices and improvement strategies. Panelists said that it would be useful to extract and compile lessons learned from providers about best practices they have implemented and to widely disseminate this information. Some panelists recommended that HHS should conduct case studies of high-performing providers to see what factors they identify as contributing to producing positive results; however, because high performers may be doing many of the same things as low performers, it is necessary to look at both high and low performers to see what differentiates them.

Alternative approaches to disseminating best practices were discussed by the TEP. Some TEP members felt that for dissemination to be effective, awareness is necessary of how low-performing organizations/providers with different resources and capabilities than the high performers will interpret and use the information that is being disseminated. Some providers may be more receptive to the information if the provider is "like them," and benefit from peer-to-peer coaching by providers located in their own community who have similar characteristics to overcome resistance to adoption of certain practices. Other providers who are willing to innovate may look to other organizations for their "good ideas" as a way to continue to improve, regardless of where they are located or their characteristics, and will embrace best practices from dissimilar organizations or practices.

Monitoring and Evaluation of Value-Based Purchasing Programs

Qualitative Evaluation

The TEP broadly agreed that there is a need for qualitative research to understand what has been learned by those who design and sponsor VBP programs and by the providers who are targets of the VBP programs. There has been a lot of iterative work by VBP program sponsors, and case studies could shed light on lessons learned that are not making their way into the published literature. Qualitative research focused on understanding what does and does not work regarding design and implementation would be useful to those designing VBP programs. For example, it would be useful to learn how providers have used performance benchmarking data provided by both public and private VBP programs to inform their quality improvement efforts and engage leadership in organizational infrastructure investments to support high-value care. One TEP member suggested Qualitative Comparative Analysis[110, 111] as one qualitative analytic methodology that might be a good fit for VBP evaluations, as it attempts to isolate key factors that are necessary conditions, versus those that are sufficient conditions, to achieve the outcome. This approach acknowledges that there are a number of possible paths or combinations of elements (e.g., alternative designs) that may lead to the desired outcome. The other area flagged by the TEP where qualitative work would be beneficial is understanding what changes providers are making in response to VBP programs. Although the TEP emphasized the need for qualitative evaluation work, there may be challenges in getting private VBP sponsors to share proprietary information, particularly in a competitive marketplace.

Quantitative Assessment of Impacts

The TEP supported the need to evaluate the impact of VBP programs, and panelists felt that having a common set of variables that potentially influence outcomes, such as program characteristics (e.g., size and type of incentives), market characteristics (e.g., extent of monopoly power among providers in the market), provider characteristics, and other facilitators/enablers, would facilitate this work. They also noted the importance of having a comparison group, as reflected by one TEP member's comment: "We need to avoid marketing techniques that claim to achieve reduction in trends when the trends were happening anyway." A comparison group guards against this possibility.

CHAPTER FOUR

Recommendations for Value-Based Purchasing Programs

Based on the findings from the environmental scan, literature review, and TEP discussions, we provide a set of recommendations for consideration that could serve to advance the design, implementation, monitoring, and evaluation of VBP programs to generate critically needed knowledge to guide policymaking. Table 2 contains the full set of recommendations. The recommendations are directed toward VBP program sponsors and the research community, both of which can play a critical role in helping to build the knowledge base.

Table 2
List of Recommendations for Value-Based Purchasing Programs

Design and Implementation of VBP Programs
1. To assess progress toward meeting goals, VBP program sponsors should consider performance targets (i.e., measurable goals) using national benchmarking data and assess progress toward meeting these specified targets.
2. To minimize the likelihood of undesired behaviors, VBP programs should case-mix-adjust outcome measures, use a broad set of measures, work with providers to identify where measure construction could lead to overtreatment, and monitor the data.
3. VBP program measures should evolve from the small, narrowly focused set of process measures currently being used toward a broader set of measures that more heavily emphasize patient outcomes.
4. VBP programs sponsors should engage providers in the design and implementation of VBP programs and support provider efforts to improve.
Monitoring and Evaluation of VBP Programs
Qualitative Evaluation
5. CMS and ASPE should augment quantitative studies of programmatic impact with qualitative evaluations to extract what is being learned from private-sector VBP programs.
6. Evaluation studies should examine the type of changes and investments that providers are making in response to VBP.
7. As new models of VBP are developed, formative evaluation work should examine implementation experiences and challenges.
Impact Assessment
8. Evaluation studies to assess VBP impact should include a comparison group.
9. Evaluation studies of VBP impacts should examine spillover effects on areas of performance that are not incentivized.
10. Program monitoring and evaluation studies should focus on understanding whether VBP programs lead to undesired effects.
General Evaluation
11. VBP program sponsors should systematically collect a common set of factors (design features, contextual factors) to facilitate being able to determine what works best and under what conditions.
12. HHS should develop a structured research agenda to address important gaps in the VBP knowledge base.

We grouped the recommendations into two broad categories: (1) *design and implementation of VBP program recommendations* and (2) *monitoring and evaluation of VBP program recommendations*. The design and implementation recommendations are further organized into four categories: setting goals and measuring success; design issues; measures; and implementation issues. The "measures" category focuses on the measures that are included in the VBP program as the basis of incentives. The monitoring and evaluation recommendations are organized into three categories: qualitative evaluation, impact assessment, and general evaluation.

In the sections that follow, we discuss each recommendation, summarizing the information from our environmental scan and TEP discussions that led to the proposed recommendation.

A. Design and Implementation Recommendations

Recommendation 1. To assess progress toward meeting goals, VBP program sponsors should consider setting performance targets (i.e., measurable goals) using national benchmarking data and assess progress toward meeting these specified targets.

The environmental scan revealed that VBP program sponsors differ in the specific program goals they set and, relatedly, their ideas of success. Defining what success means in the context of *individual* VBP programs is important for being able to assess progress toward meeting goals.

To determine whether a VBP program has been successful in improving performance on the key quality and cost indicators that providers are held accountable for, TEP members emphasized the importance of having well-defined external benchmarks as one means to gauge program success. TEP members suggested that individual VBP program sponsors use HEDIS, the Consumer Assessment of Healthcare Providers and Systems survey, or the Healthy People 2010 benchmarks to set national or regional goals (i.e., targets) for what constitutes success and to then track progress toward meeting these targets. For example, CMS could peg success for physicians or Medicare Advantage plans to achievement of the 90th percentile of performance for HEDIS measures. Performance benchmarks could similarly be established for total medical expense, by pegging the growth in risk-adjusted total cost of care year-to-year to no more than "X" percent higher than the overall rate of inflation (i.e., the Consumer Price Index).

Recommendation 2. To minimize the likelihood of undesired behaviors, VBP programs should case-mix-adjust outcome measures, use a broad set of measures, work with providers to identify where measure construction could lead to overtreatment, and monitor the data.

VBP programs seek to incentivize providers to change their behavior in desired ways to improve quality and costs; however, VBP program design features, such as the measures, size of the incentive, or thresholds, could lead to undesired behaviors, depending on the program design. While few adverse effects have been found to date related to VBP interventions, policymakers and VBP program sponsors need to remain alert to the potential for unintended consequences, particularly as VBP measures shift toward provider accountability for outcomes and if incentive payments grow in size and start to represent a considerable portion of a provider's income.

Program sponsors need to carefully consider the potential opportunities for undesired behavior to occur as a function of the way the VBP program is designed and consider ways to mitigate those effects. Certain steps can be taken related to program design and explicit monitoring to discourage providers from engaging in undesired behaviors. Several examples emerged from the TEP discussion and the review of the literature:

- **Use a broad measure set** to reduce the likelihood that providers will focus narrowly on improving care for the incentivized measures (often referred to as "teaching to the test").
- **Case-mix-adjust performance measures,** particularly for outcome measures such as clinical outcomes, length of stay, and cost measures, to account for differences in patient risk factors associated with the outcome and to counter the incentive for providers to select healthier patients to succeed (often referred to as "cherry-picking").
- **Review measures with providers** prior to their implementation to determine where undesired behaviors might occur to avoid problems of overtreatment or inappropriate treatment.
- **Audit the data,** focusing on key data elements that contribute to the performance score (upcoding of risk factors or under coding of the outcome that is being measured), to guard against gaming of the data.
- **Conduct periodic surveys of patients** (particularly those who are sicker) to identify whether providers are dumping patients that are non-adherent or restricting access for sicker patient populations (i.e., increasing disparities in care).

Case-mix adjustment remains a controversial VBP program and policy decision in terms of whether and what to risk-adjust. While case-mix adjustment can be critical to the validity of a measure (e.g., adjusting for patient severity when measuring mortality outcomes) and for countering negative behaviors among providers, there is concern about using patient risk factors as an excuse for poor performance. There is general agreement that providers should deliver evidence-based care processes to all eligible patients, regardless of SES or race/ethnicity, which has led to the absence of adjustments for process measures.

To advance the ability to empirically study unintended consequences, information is required about patients and providers who are exposed to VBP interventions; however, it has proven challenging for providers and VBP program sponsors to systematically collect data for evaluation and monitoring purposes. For example, patient-level information on race, ethnicity, SES, and other characteristics of vulnerable populations is needed to determine whether VBP is either reducing or increasing disparities. Collection of such data could enable VBP sponsors to generate performance results stratified by different subgroups to understand the impact of VBP on subgroups of the population. Another potential concern is that VBP programs may de-resource providers who most need resources to invest in quality improvement and infrastructure to provide high-quality care. Data are not routinely collected or available to evaluators to discern whether VBP programs create negative consequences for certain types of providers, such as those who disproportionately care for low-income populations. Information is needed on a provider's payer mix, the socioeconomic characteristics of their patients, and the financial health of the organization to be able to study these types of effects.

Recommendation 3. VBP program measures should evolve from the small, narrowly focused set of process measures currently being used toward a broader set of measures that more heavily emphasize patient outcomes.

Several recommendations emerged from the TEP's discussions regarding the measures that are used as the basis of payment in VBP programs. Decisions about whether and how to implement these recommendations will need to consider the resources required to develop performance measures and the burden to providers and VBP sponsors of collecting and verifying the data.

3a. Expand the measures in VBP to incentivize broad improvement. Many members of the TEP viewed applying a larger, more comprehensive set of measures in VBP programs as a way to create incentives for providers to perform well across the board and minimize the likelihood that providers will narrowly focus their improvement efforts. They held the opinion that a broad set of measures would drive wholesale quality improvement and ensure faster progress toward reaching the three aims of the National Quality Strategy. One TEP member's comment reveals the spirit of this discussion regarding the need to expand measures: "We need to say to providers, 'Here are 500 measures. We [meaning VBP sponsor/payers/purchasers] are going to pick some things from the huge list, but we want you to be good across the board.'"

Two questions are important related to measure expansion: "How much is enough?" and "What is actually feasible?" Neither the literature nor the TEP addressed how many measures are reasonable or practical to implement. Future efforts to expand the measures will need to carefully consider what constitutes the ideal set of measures to achieve the objective of incentivizing broad improvements while balancing burdens to providers of collecting and reporting the data. Policymakers must also consider the feasibility of developing a large set of measures that are valid and reliable. Given the expected difficulties associated with developing valid and reliable performance measures and the burden to providers associated with capturing and reporting the data, it seems unrealistic that VBP programs sponsors would be able to implement and hold providers accountable for 500 measures. Although 500 measures is unlikely to be the right number, we agree with the TEP that there is a need to expand our ability to more comprehensively measure the care that is provided and establish more wholesale accountabilities to raise the performance of the U.S. health system.

3b. Build the next generation of measures. Expanding the measures used in VBP programs flagged the need to develop the next generation of measures and measurement strategies. The TEP emphasized that work must begin now to build the next generation of performance measures to achieve the goals of VBP, and that CMS and the Office of the National Coordinator for Health Information Technology will need to play a leadership role in advancing measure development.

3c. Increase accountability for outcomes. The TEP members agreed that the ultimate objective of VBP is to eventually be able to hold providers accountable for their performance and financially incentivize them to improve based on measures of health outcomes. The TEP recommended that CMS work to capture functional status, which they saw as feasible (as there are existing measures for some procedures, such as shoulder, knee, and hip replacement survey) and attainable in a five-year horizon. Doing so will help shift the focus of measurement and accountability toward outcomes. The UK's National Health Service was mentioned as an example of a large health system that is successfully using broad-scale measurement of patient-reported outcomes (using the PROMs) and that may offer lessons for the United States. Additional work is required to move measures that have been tested in research contexts, such as the PROMs, to market. While we agree that efforts to advance measurement of outcomes is important, absent improved data systems to facilitate the capture of outcomes data, the feasibility of routinely capturing and reporting outcomes will prove challenging in the near term. Additionally, developing valid, reliable outcome measures that are linked to evidence-based processes and that can be proximally related to actions the providers has taken (i.e., less than one year from receipt of the process intervention) will be a significant challenge to advancing the use of outcome measures.

3d. Have a balanced portfolio of measures. VBP programs should have a balanced portfolio of measures (i.e., cost, quality, and patient experience) that includes a mix of measures that assess process, structure (e.g., intensive care unit staffing, use of computerized physician order entry systems), and outcomes. The TEP supported placing more weight on outcome measures as opposed to clinical process measures. Panelists viewed the use of process measures as an actionable tool in a stepwise progression of measurement toward measuring outcomes.

While there is concern about measures being topped out and the need for new measures, the TEP noted that there remains enormous potential for improvement on process and intermediate outcome measures in the ambulatory setting; as such, VBP programs should not shy away from using existing process and intermediate outcome measures. TEP members stated that a desired outcome is having evidence-based care processes reliably occur, and they wondered how best to maintain high performance on process measures once achieved.

3e. Measure and incentivize infrastructure investments. There was widespread agreement among the TEP that it is important to incentivize and help providers build the infrastructure for quality improvement. Systems improvement and capacity-building pieces—such as building registries to track population health, team-based care, willingness to change, and panel management—were seen as important to enabling performance improvement, and VBP programs could incentivize these structural investments. Panelists commented that the structural measures used in VBP need to be linked to improved delivery of processes and outcomes. The TEP recommended that, prior to measuring provider performance on outcomes, HHS should begin assessing provider capacity to measure patient outcomes through structural measures.

Another example of infrastructure that the TEP highlighted as important for supporting quality improvement is a provider's capacity for measuring and monitoring its own performance. Panelists commented that the Office of the National Coordinator for Health Information Technology's meaningful use requirements for certified EHRs could require that EHRs enable a data-driven environment of care delivery, as assessed by having real-time, accessible patient data for decisionmaking and proactive management of patients. Meaningful use requirements also should require that certified EHRs be able to easily generate performance measures by the provider, which, at this stage, remains very difficult and hinders the ability of providers to track their own performance.

3f. Tailor the performance measures used to meet providers where they are. Although the TEP discussion about moving to the next generation of measures emphasized tracking outcomes and that providers who have been engaged in various VBP efforts over the past decade may be ready for this kind of transition, there was recognition that not all providers are ready to move to the next generation of measures, which require more experience with measurement. The reality on the ground is that providers are at differing levels in their capabilities to respond to VBP, and the measures deployed in VBP programs need to be tailored accordingly.

Several TEP members remarked that the past decade of P4P measurement was a warm-up for many providers. Based on their experience, P4P creates a foundation for measurement and represents the first stage of getting providers to accept measurement. For the providers who have little or no experience with quality measures and are new to VBP, the TEP recommended starting with existing clinical process measures, so that providers can gain experience with data collection, being measured and held accountable, benchmarking their performance, and understanding what good performance looks like.

We agree that a strategy of using different types of measures depending on provider capabilities may facilitate engagement of all providers in VBP, which is a desired goal. However, this can create complexity for VBP program sponsors when comparing the performance of providers who are using different mixes of measures, particularly if they evaluate performance on a relative basis. One possible solution is that VBP program sponsors could establish absolute performance targets for each measure to gauge and reward provider performance. Another potential concern is that the use of different mixes of measures among providers may raise fairness concerns, as some measures may be more difficult than others for providers to achieve high performance on, putting providers on an uneven playing field related to earning incentives.

3g. Include appropriateness measures. TEP members were supportive of including measures of appropriateness (i.e., potential overuse), but recognized that additional work is required to develop the criteria and engage providers in use of these measures. In going down this path, TEP members recommended that appropriateness guidelines be created with the input from providers, in order to avoid pushback.

Recommendation 4. VBP program sponsors should engage providers in the design and implementation of VBP programs and support provider efforts to improve.

There is little in the published literature about the mechanics of program implementation and what elements are required to successfully support providers in working toward achieving the VBP program goals. The TEP provided important insights on this issue based on their experience implementing or participating in VBP programs. Provider engagement and buy-in was viewed by the TEP as critical to garnering the desired response to the incentives. The TEP recommended two ways in which the providers can be engaged.

4a. Involve providers in measure selection. The TEP emphasized that for there to be buy-in, providers need to feel comfortable that there is a relationship between measures that are the basis for payment in the VBP program and what physicians believe represents good care that will positively impact patient outcomes (i.e., evidence-based measures that are clinically compelling). The TEP also indicated that measures need to be viewed as feasible from the provider's perspective, and the actions needed to influence the measure are within the provider's locus of control. Furthermore, as noted previously, provider involvement in measure selection can help identify potential unintended consequences early on in the process.

4b. Provide support to providers to help them succeed. TEP members indicated that VBP program sponsors can engage providers in a partnership to achieve the goals of the VBP program through the provision of technical assistance to providers to help them improve. Examples of technical assistance mentioned by TEP members included providing comparative benchmarking data on variations in practice and factors contributing to differences (e.g., greater use of name brand drugs, higher use of costly imaging), infrastructure support, relevant and timely patient clinical data to facilitate care management, quality improvement support and coaching, and additional staffing support, such as care managers. CMS commented that they received many requests for data from providers in the Physician Group Practice demonstration and now in the ACO demonstrations, to help them better manage care delivery.

B. Monitoring and Evaluation Recommendations

While a variety of monitoring and evaluation studies have been conducted over the past decade related to implementation of P4P experiments, the evidence base is generally insufficient to guide policymaking related to many aspects of VBP. This research has been difficult to carry out for a number of reasons, including the challenges of conducting evaluations in observational settings and the difficulty with gaining the cooperation of VBP sponsors to have their programs evaluated and results published outside their organization. Absent cooperation by research sponsors to participate in efforts to gather and disseminate the evidence, it is likely that the VBP community will continue to muddle along as it has for much of the past decade.

To help advance the knowledge base, we offer several recommendations related to VBP program monitoring and evaluation.

Qualitative Evaluation

> **Recommendation 5.** CMS and ASPE should augment quantitative studies of programmatic impact with qualitative evaluations to extract what is being learned from private-sector VBP programs.

Although the published literature provides some insights on the impact of VBP programs in driving improvements in performance measures, it is lacking in critical information regarding specific design features, other predisposing or enabling factors that are associated with positive/negative effects, and how and why VBP programs have evolved over time. The TEP strongly endorsed the need for qualitative assessment of VBP programs to supplement quantitative impact assessments. Much has been learned through trial and error in the private sector that could inform federal efforts regarding VBP program design and implementation. VBP program sponsors tend to evolve their program designs in response to what has been learned, and this information typically is not collected, documented, and disseminated in a systematic fashion.

TEP members thought that a key advantage of qualitative work was that it could occur and generate findings more rapidly than longitudinal studies of impact. Although this may be true if the evaluation work is privately funded, we caution that any federally funded qualitative study that has more than nine study subjects would require review and approval under the Paper Reduction Act (PRA), which can be a lengthy process. We also note that another potential challenge is the proprietary nature of the information and the willingness of VBP sponsors to disclose key design elements of and lessons from their incentive programs. While some private-sector VBP sponsors may be reluctant to share information, other VBP sponsors have been more open to sharing what they have learned, and these organizations offer near-term opportunities for gathering qualitative information.

Recommendation 6. Evaluation studies should examine the type of changes and investments that providers are making in response to VBP.

Evaluation studies that examine the range and type of changes that providers are making in response to VBP could shed light on what actions providers are taking to address underlying problems with the quality and cost of care. Assessments should stratify on key variables likely to influence the ability of providers to make investments, such as size and payer mix.

Recommendation 7. As new models of VBP are developed, formative evaluation work should examine implementation experiences and challenges.

Documenting what is learned in the process of designing and implementing new VBP models (i.e., ACOs, bundled payments) will be beneficial to those testing the models and to policymakers, who will want to learn how to scale these models if they are found to be successful. Because these models are still in their early stage of development, much can be learned by conducting formative evaluations to understand factors that help or hinder the functioning of these models, the types of relationships that are being established between different providers (e.g., ambulatory providers and hospitals) and between providers and payers within these arrangements, the extent of support required by payers (e.g., providing data for real-time patient management), the amount and type of risk being borne by providers, the role of HIT in enabling these care delivery models to function and achieve goals, where the provider organizations are making structural investments to support achievement of goals, and the extent of communication across providers and how this has changed as a function of the new performance-based payment model. Qualitative assessments could be a useful tool to gather information on the design and functioning of these new VBP models.

Impact Assessment

> **Recommendation 8.** Evaluation studies to assess VBP impact should include a comparison group.

A large share of the P4P evaluations over the past decade lacked comparison groups that would allow evaluators to disentangle the P4P effects from other interventions that were also in play to address the problems of poor quality and high costs. Because of the substantial cost and administrative burdens that VBP programs involve for both program sponsors and providers, it is important that policymakers understand whether the investment of resources they are making in VBP is having impact. If they are not, then resources can be deployed to other interventions that may have more impact in improving quality and value.

The TEP members agreed that impact studies should have a comparison group to control for confounding factors that may explain observed outcomes. While comparison groups may not be feasible in all situations—such as when VBP policies are rolled out nationally—policymakers will need to be careful in interpreting the results of such studies to gauge whether observed effects would have likely occurred absent the intervention. As stated earlier in this report, this is why it is especially important that evaluators conducting observational studies select theory-driven hypotheses about how incentives affect behavior, so as to identify potential confounding factors that could explain observed effects.[18]

> **Recommendation 9.** Evaluation studies of VBP impacts should examine spillover effects on areas of performance that are not incentivized.

The published evidence on spillover effects is very limited and inconclusive. There is currently insufficient evidence to determine whether VBP programs have spillover effects and where effects occur. Evaluation of spillover effects has proven challenging, because in many cases, data on other "non-incentivized" measures or patient populations were not collected or available for comparison. The TEP recommended, and we concur, that CMS and private VBP sponsors conduct evaluation work to assess spillover effects on cost, utilization, and quality.

> **Recommendation 10.** Program monitoring and evaluation studies should focus on understanding whether VBP programs lead to undesired effects.

While studies of P4P programs and bundled payments have not found much in the way of adverse effects, it remains very important for VBP programs to monitor for potential undesired effects: As changes to the types of measures and the size and design of the incentives occur, the incentives for undesired behavior may increase. For example, as programs shift to outcome measures, this may adversely affect providers who care for more challenging patient populations, where achieving a high level of performance may prove more difficult. The TEP strongly supported monitoring and evaluation work to understand whether VBP programs result in unintended effects, including the following:

- **Assess changes in market concentration and the impacts on prices, particularly in the context of newer VBP models.** ACO and bundled payment models are sparking greater integration and consolidation in markets, and it is unclear whether this may lead to reduced competition and higher prices.
- **Monitor patient experience, access to care, and patient turnover from practices to assess whether providers are avoiding caring for more difficult patients.** Surveys of patients and analyses of utilization and case-mix data can be used to understand whether providers are avoiding caring for more difficult patients. These efforts could be supplemented with surveys of providers to understand whether they are engaging in such practices and what could be done to mitigate this problem. TEP members flagged the importance of collecting SES, race/ethnicity, health literacy, and self-reported literacy data in order to understand changes in disparities; however, they expressed skepticism about the ability to measure and report on many of these variables.
- **Explore how VBP is impacting care delivered for non-incentivized areas to understand whether unmeasured areas suffer.** This will require that organizations track performance on non-incentivized measures or conduct periodic reviews of claims or medical record data to understand impacts on areas of care that are not the focus of the incentive program.
- **Assess the distribution of VBP payments (winners and losers), particularly how it affects providers who care for more challenging patient populations and may have fewer resources to respond to VBP.** There is interest in increasing the size of incentives to generate greater impact. VBP program sponsors should monitor the distribution of incentive payments to understand whether VBP programs de-resource the subset of providers who most need to invest in infrastructure, process re-engineering, and staffing to raise poor performance.
- **Monitoring for inappropriate or overtreatment.** Commonly used measures that set dichotomous targets (i.e., meet or do not meet a threshold, such as HbA1c less than 7) can create incentives for providers to get all patients to the threshold, whether or not it is clinically appropriate or in keeping with patient preferences. Studies should monitor the extent to which this may be occurring to spotlight problems with measures so that the measures used in VBP programs can be redesigned to mitigate these effects.

General Evaluation

> **Recommendation 11.** VBP program sponsors should systematically collect a common set of factors (design features, contextual factors) to facilitate being able to determine what works best and under what conditions.

The ability to synthesize the lessons learned from the studies of the past decade has been handicapped by the lack of a uniform set of factors that may be important predictors of VBP program success or, instead, confounding factors. A common catalog of VBP program characteristics (design features, contextual factors) was viewed by the TEP as necessary to determine whether we are studying the same thing or different things when comparing across studies. The value of having a common set of variables across all programs is that it can facilitate a more synthetic approach to evaluating VBP programs. Currently, each VBP program is assessed separately to find effects rather than looking across different VBP programs to see how specific measures that are common across programs have improved or how different incentive structures drive improvement. The TEP stated that an "across program" synthesis of what has been learned is needed to inform under what conditions VBP works.

The appendix to this report contains a candidate list of variables identified in our discussions with the TEP. Given constraints in the number of data elements that could be reasonably collected, we believe an important next step is for CMS and other federal agencies with a VBP role to work with private-sector VBP sponsors and researchers to identify the high-priority variables and the way in which these variables should be commonly coded across programs. This step could also include agreement among private and public stakeholders to collect these variables. Systematic collection of the variables for all VBP programs would be an important step toward facilitating program evaluations and the ability to compare and contrast observed impacts across programs. Federal agencies have the ability to make collection of these variables a condition of receipt of federal funding—such as in the context of the Center for Medicare and Medicaid Innovation's grants for testing new models of care delivery and VBP, such as ACOs.

Recommendation 12. HHS should develop a structured research agenda to address important gaps in the VBP knowledge base.

It is vital that the VBP community (i.e., program sponsors, providers, researchers, and policymakers) embrace a well-specified and prioritized research agenda so that scarce evaluation resources can be best deployed to generate the information needed to guide policymaking. Among the knowledge gap areas that emerged from our review and discussions with the TEP were the following:

- **What is the impact of different incentive structures on VBP success, and how should incentives be structured to elicit desired behavioral responses?** There are a variety of VBP incentive structures being tested, and it would be useful to understand the impacts that alternative incentive structures have on driving improvement. This includes: How large do incentives need to be to drive the desired changes? What types of measures should be used? Do provider responses to incentive structures differ based on the type of structure used (e.g., fixed thresholds, improvement and attainment, relative performance)? Should all providers have the same incentive to motivate behavior change? It is unclear whether incentives targeted at the organization level are pushed down to front-line providers aligned with the organization's incentives. Is VBP success influenced by the type of incentives that front-line physicians face?
- **What is the impact of VBP programs? In what contexts is improvement occurring?** Provider organizations and the markets in which they operate are heterogeneous, and there is poor understanding of how these contextual factors influence improvement efforts. Little is known about whether some types of measures work better in driving

improvement than others; as VBP advances toward the inclusion of more outcome measures, it will be important to evaluate whether they stimulate greater improvements in quality and value. If measured areas are lagging in performance, why, and could program design and implementation be modified to affect performance in lagging areas? How do VBP programs affect provider satisfaction and experiences? What is the effect of VBP programs on local health care markets (e.g., provider consolidation, increased integration of hospitals and physician practices)?

- **What are the behavioral and system responses to VBP programs?** Understanding whether VBP incentivizes providers to build capacity and infrastructure and to redesign care delivery is essential for knowing what actions VBP prompts and whether these actions help drive improvements. Also, how do different types of providers (high- versus low-performing) respond?
- **What differentiates high and low performers under VBP programs?** There is limited evidence on what characterizes high and low performers under incentive schemes. Such information could be useful for shedding light on the types of infrastructure and other features that need to be in place to succeed, and to find ways of embedding those elements among low performing providers.
- **To what extent do VBP programs lead to unintended consequences?** As incentives grow in size and the measures evolve toward outcomes where providers will face increased difficulty achieving the measures, it is important to continually monitor for undesired effects.
- **To what extent do VBP programs facilitate broad improvements in quality by creating spillover effects?** As VBP programs continue to evolve and other design elements are embedded (e.g., risk sharing, incentives for integration, investments in infrastructure), it is important to know the broader effects that result from the changes that providers are making in response to VBP. Do these investments lead organizations to perform well across the board?
- **How important is public reporting as an incentive, as compared with the use of financial incentives?** A primary motivator for change likely has been transparency, in part, because the financial incentives in P4P have been relatively small to date. Determining the relative importance of public reporting versus financial incentives in driving improvements has implications for program sponsors, who are expending substantial resources in computing incentive payouts and managing these programs.

CHAPTER FIVE

Conclusion

The application of performance-based payment models represents a work in progress regarding how best to design VBP programs to achieve desired goals, the optimal conditions that support successful implementation, and provider response to the incentives. We believe that continued innovation is desired at this early stage of VBP development and implementation. Concerted efforts will be required to ensure that the lessons learned from these experiments are identified and disseminated to advance the use of VBP as a strategy for improving federal and private health care programs.

From this review, we identify three critical areas that require attention to advance progress on the federal government's use of VBP as a strategy for driving improvements in the health system:

1. **Develop a National Value-Based Purchasing Strategy.** HHS should develop a national VBP strategy for Medicare analogous to its National Quality Strategy. HHS should form a workgroup that brings together representatives from CMS, ASPE, AHRQ, and other government agencies and draws on the expertise of private-sector program sponsors and providers to develop the strategy. The strategy should outline what the federal government's goals are for VBP and thus what constitutes success, the priority areas for measurement, a timeline for increased focus on outcomes and other high-priority measurement areas, and a coordinated research agenda across CMS's VBP initiatives. The strategy will also need to consider the interplay between various CMS VBP initiatives in working to advance federal goals for VBP and how those initiatives could better align incentives to providers.
2. **Develop a Well-Defined, Coordinated Research Strategy.** Many unanswered questions remain about VBP's effectiveness and the features associated with successful VBP programs. How and why VBP programs do or do not work are very complicated questions. A well-defined, coordinated research strategy is needed to generate the information required to fill gaps in the knowledge base. Currently, federal efforts to develop, test, and evaluate VBP programs are occurring setting by setting. This presents an opportunity to coordinate the evaluation work being performed across the various VBP initiatives within CMS to draw lessons across programs and provider settings that will inform the design and implementation of the next phase of VBP programs. As a first step, HHS could work to develop a common evaluation framework and a prioritized set of research questions, by setting and across settings, that would serve to guide CMS-sponsored evaluation studies, better align the actions of the agency to generate the desired knowledge, and coordinate use of limited evaluation resources.

The systematic collection of a core set of program design and context variables for all VBP programs would be an important step toward facilitating program evaluations and the ability to compare and contrast observed impacts across programs. Federal agencies have the ability to make collection of these variables a condition of receipt of federal funding—such as in the context of the Center for Medicare and Medicaid Innovation's grants for testing new models of care delivery and VBP, such as ACOs. HHS and CMS should leverage Medicare and Medicaid reporting requirements and HHS-sponsored experiments to learn more than we know today. Additionally, HHS could support the formation of a private/public-sector learning collaborative, with participating organizations agreeing to share design information and other data with researchers, using an agreed-upon data sharing protocol and participating in the development of the research questions.

3. **Chart a New Strategy and Process for Developing Measures to Support Federal Value-Based Purchasing Programs.** Performance measures are foundational to VBP. The heavy emphasis on performance measures in the TEP discussions underscores the importance of measures to the VBP enterprise and the inadequacy of existing performance measures to transform the delivery of health care. Progress to develop a new generation of performance measures should be accelerated and streamlined to meet the urgent and growing needs of the VBP programs to move beyond primarily assessing processes of care to also focus on evaluating patient outcomes and the appropriate use of services. We encourage ASPE to work with measure-development experts to chart a new strategy and process for developing measures to support VBP programs.

APPENDIX

Program Design and Context Variables

VBP Approaches and Program Design Features

- Structure of incentive
  - Frequency (e.g., annual, per service)
  - Magnitude (revenue potential)
  - Type of incentive (e.g., bonus, increase on fee-for-service/per diem/DRG payment, penalty, public reporting of performance, shared savings, upside/downside risk)
    - Use of non-financial incentives
    - Form of financing (e.g., withhold, new dollars, based on savings)
  - Types of benchmarks/thresholds
    - Absolute performance (percentile ranking or fixed threshold)
    - Relative performance
      - Improvement (continuous)
  - Target of the incentive
- Measures
  - Number of measures
  - Types of measures (structure, process, outcomes; cost or quality)
    - Difficulty of measure (to achieve success)—does it require patient cooperation?
    - Perceived attainability (is performance within the provider's control?)
  - Baseline performance on chosen measures
    - Use of risk/case-mix adjustment (and adjusted for what factors?)
    - Attribution method
- Sponsor of the incentive (plan, purchaser, medical group)
- Technical support provided by VBP sponsor
  - Data transparency with providers (variations analyses)/use of performance feedback
  - Case management and care coordination resources
  - Sharing of best practices/learning networks
  - Coaching/training
  - Other technical assistance
- Overall approach to paying for services (base payment model on which the VBP program operates)— fee-for-service, capitation, global payment (hospital and physician), bundled payment
  - Consumer incentives and engagement strategies

Characteristics of the Providers and Practice Settings

- Populations served (payer mix, patient characteristics including socioeconomic mix, insurance status, age, clinical conditions)
- Incentive mix at different levels of the provider organization (capitation, salary, fee-for-service)
- Extent to which provider network is restricted
- Size of the provider (i.e., number of beds, number of patients in panel)
- Percentage of provider's patients for whom the incentive is relevant
- Organization structure/ type (e.g., integrated medical group, independent practice association, primary care practice site, medical home, etc.)
- Organizational culture, leadership
- Use of peer pressure
- Extent of provider integration within a delivery system
- Health information technology use (extent, types)
- Other incentives faced by the provider (e.g., for utilization) and magnitude of those incentives
- Cost of compliance/improving quality (versus the incentives offered)
- Clinician characteristics (e.g., specialties, age, gender)
- Use of guidelines by provider
- Participation in external quality improvement collaboratives

Other External Factors

- Market characteristics (e.g., market concentration/competitiveness, number of payers, market share of each payer)
- Exposure to other VBP programs and quality initiatives across payers in a market (mix of incentives in the market)
- Alignment of measures across VBP programs within a market
- Regulatory features
- Anticipation of future policy trends (momentum regarding the inevitability of VBP)

References

1. Damberg CL, Sorbero ME, Mehrotra A, Teleki S, Lovejoy S, Bradley L. An Environmental Scan of Pay for Performance in the Hospital Setting: Final Report. Washington, DC: Office of the Assistant Secretary for Planning and Evaluation (ASPE). 2007.

2. Rosenthal MB, de Brantes FS, Sinaiko AD, Frankel M, Robbins RD, Young S. Bridges to excellence—recognizing high-quality care: Analysis of physician quality and resource use. American Journal of Managed Care. 2008 Oct;14(10):670–677.

3. Sorbero MES, Damberg CL, Shaw R, Teleki S, Lovejoy S, Decristofaro A, Dembosky J, Schuster C. Assessment of Pay-for-Performance Options for Medicare Physician Services: Final Report. Santa Monica, CA: RAND Corporation. WR-391-ASPE. 2006. As of November 20, 2013: http://www.rand.org/pubs/working_papers/WR391.html

4. Curtin K, Beckman H, Pankow G, Milillo Y, Green RA. Return on investment in pay for performance: A diabetes case study. Journal of Healthcare Management. 2006 Nov–Dec;51(6):365–74; discussion 75–76.

5. Damberg CL, Raube K, Teleki SS, Dela Cruz E. Taking stock of pay-for-performance: A candid assessment from the front lines. Health Affairs (Millwood). 2009 Mar–Apr;28(2):517–525.

6. Pearson SD, Schneider EC, Kleinman KP, Coltin KL, Singer JA. The impact of pay-for-performance on health care quality in Massachusetts, 2001–2003. Health Affairs. 2008 Jul–Aug;27(4):1167–1176.

7. Stecher BM, Camm F, Damberg CL, Hamilton LS, Mullen KJ, Nelson C, Sorensen P, Wachs M, Yoh A, Zellman GL, Leuschner KJ. Toward a Culture of Consequences: Performance-Based Accountability Systems for Public Services. Santa Monica, CA: RAND Corporation. MG-1019. 2010. As of November 20, 2013: http://www.rand.org/pubs/monographs/MG1019.html

8. Damberg CL, Shortell SM, Raube K, Gillies RR, Rittenhouse D, McCurdy RK, Casalino LP, Adams J. Relationship between quality improvement processes and clinical performance. American Journal of Managed Care. 2010 Aug;16(8):601–606.

9. Young GJ, Meterko M, Beckman H, Baker E, White B, Sautter KM, Greene R, Curtin K, Bokhour BG, Berlowitz D, Burgess JF, Jr. Effects of paying physicians based on their relative performance for quality. Journal of General Internal Medicine. 2007 Jun;22(6):872–876.

10. Christianson JB, Leatherman S, Sutherland K. Lessons from evaluations of purchaser pay-for-performance programs: A review of the evidence. Medical Care Research and Review. 2008 Dec;65(6 Suppl):5S–35S.

11. Rosenthal MB, Frank RG, Li Z, Epstein AM. Early experience with pay-for-performance: from concept to practice. JAMA. 2005 Oct 12;294(14):1788–1793.

12. Hussey PS, Sorbero ME, Mehrotra A, Liu H, Damberg CL. Episode-based performance measurement and payment: Making it a reality. Health Affairs. 2009 Sep-Oct;28(5):1406–1417.

13. Hussey PS, Mulcahy AW, Schnyer C, Schneider EC. Bundled payment: Effects on health care spending and quality. Rockville, MD: Agency for Healthcare Research and Quality. 2012.

14. Hussey PS, Ridgely MS, Rosenthal MB. The PROMETHEUS bundled payment experiment: Slow start shows problems in implementing new payment models. Health Affairs. 2011 Nov;30(11):2116–2124.

15. 111th United States Congress. Patient Protection and Affordable Care Act Pub.L. 111-148. Washington, DC. 2010.

16. National Quality Strategy. [cited 2013 July 15]. As of November 5, 2013: http://www.ahrq.gov/workingforquality/reports.htm

17. U.S. Department of Health and Human Service. 2012 Annual Progress Report to Congress. National Strategy for Quality Improvement in Health Care. Washington, DC: U.S. Department of Health and Human Services. April 2012 (Corrected August 2012).

18. Dudley RA. Pay-for-performance research: How to learn what clinicians and policy makers need to know. JAMA. 2005 Oct 12;294(14):1821–1823.

19. Dudley RA, Frolich A, Robinowitz DL, Talavera JA, Broadhead P, Luft HS. Strategies to support quality-based purchasing: A review of the evidence. Technical Review 10. (Prepared by the Stanford-University of California San Francisco Evidence-based Practice Center under Contract No. 290-02-0017.) AHRQ Publication No. 04-0057. Rockville, MD: Agency for Healthcare Research and Quality. 2004 Jul.

20. McHugh M, Joshi M. Improving evaluations of value-based purchasing programs. Health Services Research. 2010 Oct;45(5 Pt 2):1559–1569.

21. Fisher ES, Shortell SM, Kreindler SA, Van Citters AD, Larson BK. A framework for evaluating the formation, implementation, and performance of accountable care organizations. Health Affairs. 2012 Nov;31(11):2368–2378.

22. Damberg CL, Sorbero ME, Lovejoy S, Martsolf GR, Raaen L, Mandel D. Measuring Success in Healthcare Value-Based Purchasing Programs: Findings from an Environmental Scan, Literature Review, and Expert Panel Discussions. Santa Monica, CA: RAND Corporation. RR-306-ASPE. 2013.

23. McGlynn EA, Asch SM, Adams J, Keesey J, Hicks J, DeCristofaro A, Kerr EA. The quality of health care delivered to adults in the United States. New England Journal of Medicine. 2003 Jun 26;348(26):2635–2645.

24. Centers for Medicare and Medicaid Services. National Provider Call: Hospital Value-Based Purchasing: Fiscal Year 2015 Overview for Beneficiaries, Providers, and Stakeholders. Baltimore, MD: Centers for Medicare and Medicaid Services. 2013.

25. Health Services Advisory Group. Is Your Hospital Ready for Value-Based Purchasing? Phoenix, AZ: Health Services Advisory Group. 2013 [cited 2013 November 4]. As of November 5, 2013:
http://www.hsag.com/App_Resources/Documents/VBP_factsheet_-FLCA_508.pdf

26. Tak HJ, Ruhnke GW, Meltzer DO. Association of patient preferences for participation in decision making with length of stay and costs among hospitalized patients. JAMA Internal Medicine. 2013 Jul 8;173(13):1195–1205.

27. Doran T, Fullwood C, Reeves D, Gravelle H, Roland M. Exclusion of patients from pay-for-performance targets by English physicians. New England Journal of Medicine. 2008 Jul 17;359(3):274–284.

28. Chien AT, Li Z, Rosenthal MB. Improving timely childhood immunizations through pay for performance in Medicaid-managed care. Health Services Research. 2010 Dec;45(6 Pt 2):1934–1947.

29. Fairbrother G, Siegel MJ, Friedman S, Kory PD, Butts GC. Impact of financial incentives on documented immunization rates in the inner city: Results of a randomized controlled trial. Ambulatory Pediatrics. 2001 Jul–Aug;1(4):206–212.

30. Serumaga B, Ross-Degnan D, Avery AJ, Elliott RA, Majumdar SR, Zhang F, Soumerai SB. Effect of pay for performance on the management and outcomes of hypertension in the United Kingdom: interrupted time series study. British Medical Journal. 2011;342:d108.

31. Gilmore AS, Zhao Y, Kang N, Ryskina KL, Legorreta AP, Taira DA, Chung RS. Patient outcomes and evidence-based medicine in a preferred provider organization setting: a six-year evaluation of a physician pay-for-performance program. Health Services Research. 2007 Dec;42(6 Pt 1):2140–2159; discussion 294–323.

32. Chung RS, Chernicoff HO, Nakao KA, Nickel RC, Legorreta AP. A quality-driven physician compensation model: four-year follow-up study. Journal for Healthcare Quality. 2003 Nov–Dec;25(6):31–37.

33. Coleman K, Reiter KL, Fulwiler D. The impact of pay-for-performance on diabetes care in a large network of community health centers. Journal of Health Care for the Poor and Underserved. 2007 Nov;18(4):966–983.

34. Cutler TW, Palmieri J, Khalsa M, Stebbins M. Evaluation of the relationship between a chronic disease care management program and California pay-for-performance diabetes care cholesterol measures in one medical group. Journal of Managed Care Pharmacy. 2007 Sep;13(7):578–588.

35. Larsen DL, Cannon W, Towner S. Longitudinal assessment of a diabetes care management system in an integrated health network. Journal of Managed Care Pharmacy. 2003;9(6):552–558.

36. Amundson G, Solberg LI, Reed M, Martini EM, Carlson R. Paying for quality improvement: compliance with tobacco cessation guidelines. Joint Commission Journal on Quality and Patient Safety. 2003 Feb;29(2):59–65.

37. Hung DY, Green LA. Paying for prevention: associations between pay for performance and cessation counseling in primary care practices. American Journal of Health Promotion. 2012 Mar–Apr;26(4):230–234.

38. Armour BS, Friedman C, Pitts MM, Wike J, Alley L, Etchason J. The influence of year-end bonuses on colorectal cancer screening. American Journal of Managed Care. 2004 Sep;10(9):617–624.

39. Chung S, Palaniappan LP, Trujillo LM, Rubin HR, Luft HS. Effect of physician-specific pay-for-performance incentives in a large group practice. American Journal of Managed Care. 2010 Feb;16(2):e35–e42.

40. Pourat N, Rice T, Tai-Seale M, Bolan G, Nihalani J. Association between physician compensation methods and delivery of guideline-concordant STD care: Is there a link? American Journal of Managed Care. 2005 Jul;11(7):426–432.

41. Greene RA, Beckman H, Chamberlain J, Partridge G, Miller M, Burden D, Kerr J. Increasing adherence to a community-based guideline for acute sinusitis through education, physician profiling, and financial incentives. American Journal of Managed Care. 2004 Oct;10(10):670–678.

42. Mandel KE, Kotagal UR. Pay for performance alone cannot drive quality. Archives of Pediatrics and Adolescent Medicine. 2007 Jul;161(7):650–655.

43. Unutzer J, Chan YF, Hafer E, Knaster J, Shields A, Powers D, Veith RC. Quality improvement with pay-for-performance incentives in integrated behavioral health care. American Journal of Public Health. 2012 Jun;102(6):e41–e45.

44. Collier VU. Use of pay for performance in a community hospital private hospitalist group: a preliminary report. Transactions of the American Clinical and Climatological Association. 2007;118:263–272.

45. Leitman IM, Levin R, Lipp MJ, Sivaprasad L, Karalakulasingam CJ, Bernard DS, Friedmann P, Shulkin DJ. Quality and financial outcomes from gainsharing for inpatient admissions: a three-year experience. Journal of Hospital Medicine. 2010 Nov–Dec;5(9):501–507.

46. Fagan PJ, Schuster AB, Boyd C, Marsteller JA, Griswold M, Murphy SM, Dunbar L, Forrest CB. Chronic care improvement in primary care: Evaluation of an integrated pay-for-performance and practice-based care coordination program among elderly patients with diabetes. Health Services Research. 2010 Dec;45(6 Pt 1):1763–1782.

47. Beaulieu ND, Horrigan DR. Putting smart money to work for quality improvement. Health Services Research. 2005 Oct;40(5 Pt 1):1318–1334.

48. Mullen KJ, Frank RG, Rosenthal MB. Can you get what you pay for? Pay-for-performance and the quality of healthcare providers. RAND Journal of Economics. 2010 Spring;41(1):64–91.

49. Chien AT, Wroblewski K, Damberg C, Williams TR, Yanagihara D, Yakunina Y, Casalino LP. Do physician organizations located in lower socioeconomic status areas score lower on pay-for-performance measures? Journal of General Internal Medicine. 2012 May;27(5):548–554.

50. Felt-Lisk S, Gimm G, Peterson S. Making pay-for-performance work in Medicaid. Health Affairs. 2007 Jul–Aug;26(4):w516–w527.

51. Levin-Scherz J, DeVita N, Timbie J. Impact of pay-for-performance contracts and network registry on diabetes and asthma HEDIS measures in an integrated delivery network. Medical Care Research and Review. 2006 Feb;63(1 Suppl):14S–28S.

52. Lester H, Schmittdiel J, Selby J, Fireman B, Campbell S, Lee J, Whippy A, Madvig P. The impact of removing financial incentives from clinical quality indicators: Longitudinal analysis of four Kaiser Permanente indicators. BMJ. 2010;340:c1898.

53. Roski J, Jeddeloh R, An L, Lando H, Hannan P, Hall C, Zhu SH. The impact of financial incentives and a patient registry on preventive care quality: Increasing provider adherence to evidence-based smoking cessation practice guidelines. Preventive Medicine. 2003 Mar;36(3):291–299.

54. Chen JY, Tian H, Taira Juarez D, Hodges KA, Jr., Brand JC, Chung RS, Legorreta AP. The effect of a PPO pay-for-performance program on patients with diabetes. American Journal of Managed Care. 2010 Jan;16(1):e11–e19.

55. An LC, Bluhm JH, Foldes SS, Alesci NL, Klatt CM, Center BA, Nersesian WS, Larson ME, Ahluwalia JS, Manley MW. A randomized trial of a pay-for-performance program targeting clinician referral to a state tobacco quitline. Archives of Internal Medicine. 2008 Oct 13;168(18):1993–1999.

56. Chen JY, Kang N, Juarez DT, Hodges KA, Chung RS, Legorreta AP. Impact of a pay-for-performance program on low performing physicians. Journal for Healthcare Quality. 2010 Jan–Feb;32(1):13–21; quiz -2.

57. Gavagan TF, Du H, Saver BG, Adams GJ, Graham DM, McCray R, Goodrick GK. Effect of financial incentives on improvement in medical quality indicators for primary care. The Journal of the American Board of Family Medicine. 2010 Sep–Oct;23(5):622–631.

58. Glickman SW, Ou FS, DeLong ER, Roe MT, Lytle BL, Mulgund J, Rumsfeld JS, Gibler WB, Ohman EM, Schulman KA, Peterson ED. Pay for performance, quality of care, and outcomes in acute myocardial infarction. JAMA. 2007 Jun 6;297(21):2373–2380.

59. Nicholas LH, Dimick JB, Iwashyna TJ. Do hospitals alter patient care effort allocations under pay-for-performance? Health Services Research. 2011 Feb;46(1 Pt 1):61–81.

60. Ryan AM, Blustein J. The effect of the MassHealth hospital pay-for-performance program on quality. Health Services Research. 2011 Jun;46(3):712–728.

61. Werner RM, Kolstad JT, Stuart EA, Polsky D. The effect of pay-for-performance in hospitals: Lessons for quality improvement. Health Affairs. 2011 Apr;30(4):690–698.

62. Calikoglu S, Murray R, Feeney D. Hospital pay-for-performance programs in Maryland produced strong results, including reduced hospital-acquired conditions. Health Affairs. 2012 Dec;31(12):2649–2658.

63. Ryan AM, Blustein J, Doran T, Michelow MD, Casalino LP. The effect of Phase 2 of the Premier Hospital Quality Incentive Demonstration on incentive payments to hospitals caring for disadvantaged patients. Health Services Research. 2012 Aug;47(4):1418–1436.

64. Lindenauer PK, Remus D, Roman S, Rothberg MB, Benjamin EM, Ma A, Bratzler DW. Public reporting and pay for performance in hospital quality improvement. New England Journal of Medicine. 2007;356(5):486–496.

65. Herrin J, Nicewander D, Ballard DJ. The effect of health care system administrator pay-for-performance on quality of care. Joint Commission Journal on Quality and Patient Safety. 2008 Nov;34(11):646–654.

66. Shepard DS, Calabro JA, Love CT, McKay JR, Tetreault J, Yeom HS. Counselor incentives to improve client retention in an outpatient substance abuse aftercare program. Administration and Policy in Mental Health. 2006 Nov;33(6):629–635.

67. Colla CH, Wennberg DE, Meara E, Skinner JS, Gottlieb D, Lewis VA, Snyder CM, Fisher ES. Spending differences associated with the Medicare Physician Group Practice Demonstration. JAMA. 2012 Sep 12;308(10):1015–1023.

68. Markovich P. A global budget pilot project among provider partners and Blue Shield of California led to savings in first two years. Health Affairs. 2012 Sep;31(9):1969–1976.

69. Salmon RB, Sanderson MI, Walters BA, Kennedy K, Flores RC, Muney AM. A collaborative accountable care model in three practices showed promising early results on costs and quality of care. Health Affairs. 2012 Nov;31(11):2379–2387.

70. Song Z, Safran DG, Landon BE, He Y, Ellis RP, Mechanic RE, Day MP, Chernew ME. Health care spending and quality in year 1 of the alternative quality contract. New England Journal of Medicine. 2011 Sep 8;365(10):909–918.

71. Song Z, Safran DG, Landon BE, Landrum MB, He Y, Mechanic RE, Day MP, Chernew ME. The "Alternative Quality Contract," based on a global budget, lowered medical spending and improved quality. Health Affairs. 2012 Aug;31(8):1885–1894.

72. Centers for Medicare and Medicaid Services. Press release: Pioneer Accountable Care Organizations succeed in improving care, lowering costs. Baltimore, MD: Centers for Medicare and Medicaid Services. 2013 [cited 2013 August 16]. As of November 5, 2013: http://www.cms.gov/Newsroom/MediaReleaseDatabase/Press-Releases/2013-Press-Releases-Items/2013-07-16.html

73. Casale AS, Paulus RA, Selna MJ, Doll MC, Bothe Jr AE, McKinley KE, Berry SA, Davis DE, Gilfillan RJ, Hamory BH. "ProvenCareSM": A provider-driven pay-for-performance program for acute episodic cardiac surgical care. Annals of Surgery. 2007;246(4):613–623.

74. Chien AT, Eastman D, Li Z, Rosenthal MB. Impact of a pay for performance program to improve diabetes care in the safety net. Preventive Medicine. 2012 Nov;55 Suppl:S80-S85.

75. Rosenthal MB, Li Z, Robertson AD, Milstein A. Impact of financial incentives for prenatal care on birth outcomes and spending. Health Services Research. 2009 Oct;44(5 Pt 1):1465–1479.

76. Ryan AM. Effects of the Premier Hospital Quality Incentive Demonstration on Medicare patient mortality and cost. Health Services Research. 2009 Jun;44(3):821–842.

77. Sutton M, Nikolova S, Boaden R, Lester H, McDonald R, Roland M. Reduced mortality with hospital pay for performance in England. New England Journal of Medicine. 2012 Nov 8;367(19):1821–1828.

78. Jha AK, Joynt KE, Orav EJ, Epstein AM. The long-term effect of premier pay for performance on patient outcomes. New England Journal of Medicine. 2012 Apr 26;366(17):1606–1615.

79. Werner RM, Rita T, Kim M. Quality improvement under nursing home compare: the association between changes in process and outcome measures. Medical care. 2013;51(7):582–588.

80. Hittle D, Nuccio E, Richard A. Evaluation of the Medicare Home Health Pay-for-Performance Demonstration: CY2008 Report—Volume 1: Agency Characteristics, Costs, and Quality Measure Performance among Treatment, Control, and Non-Participant Groups 2011.

81. Shen Y. Selection incentives in a performance-based contracting system. Health Services Research. 2003;38(2):535–552.

82. Kruse GB, Polsky D, Stuart EA, Werner RM. The impact of hospital pay-for-performance on hospital and Medicare costs. Health Services Research. 2012 Oct 22.

83. Ryan AM, Burgess JF, Jr., Tompkins CP, Wallack SS. The relationship between Medicare's process of care quality measures and mortality. Inquiry. 2009 Fall;46(3):274–290.

84. Zucker M, editor. Case Study 1: Prospective Payment for Medicare Parts A and B During Hospitalization (ACE Demo). Episode Payment: Private Innovation and Opportunities for Medicare. Washington, DC: Brandeis University. 2011.

85. Beard AJ, Hofer TP, Downs JR, Lucatorto M, Klamerus ML, Holleman R, Kerr EA. Assessing appropriateness of lipid management among patients with diabetes mellitus: moving from target to treatment. Circulation: Cardiovascular Quality and Outcomes. 2013 Jan 1;6(1):66–74.

86. Kerr EA, Hayward RA. Patient-centered performance management: enhancing value for patients and health care systems. JAMA. 2013 Jul 10;310(2):137–138.

87. Kerr EA, Lucatorto MA, Holleman R, Hogan MM, Klamerus ML, Hofer TP. Monitoring performance for blood pressure management among patients with diabetes mellitus: Too much of a good thing? Archives of Internal Medicine. 2012;172(12):938–945.

88. Friedberg MW, Mehrotra A, Linder JA. Reporting hospitals' antibiotic timing in pneumonia: adverse consequences for patients? American Journal of Managed Care. 2009 Feb;15(2):137–144.

89. Campbell B, Marchildon GP. Table of contents for Medicare: Facts, Myths, Problems, Promise: J. Lorimer & Co.; 2007 [cited WorldCat. ACO 20121106]. As of November 5, 2013:
http://catdir.loc.gov/catdir/toc/fy0803/2008360115.html

90. Campbell SM, Reeves D, Kontopantelis E, Sibbald B, Roland M. Effects of pay for performance on the quality of primary care in England. New England Journal of Medicine. 2009 Jul 23;361(4):368–378.

91. Healy D, Cromwell J. Hospital-acquired conditions—present on admission: Examination of spillover effects and unintended consequences. Baltimore, MD: Centers for Medicare and Medicaid Services. 2012.

92. McWilliams JM, Landon BE, Chernew ME. Changes in health care spending and quality for Medicare beneficiaries associated with a commercial ACO contract. JAMA. 2013 Aug 28;310(8):829–836.

93. Jha AK, Orav EJ, Epstein AM. The effect of financial incentives on hospitals that serve poor patients. Annals of Internal Medicine. 2010 Sep 7;153(5):299–306.

94. Ryan AM. Has pay-for-performance decreased access for minority patients? Health Services Research. 2010 Feb;45(1):6–23.

95. Ryan AM, Blustein J, Casalino LP. Medicare's flagship test of pay-for-performance did not spur more rapid quality improvement among low-performing hospitals. Health Affairs. 2012 Apr;31(4):797–805.

96. Doran T, Fullwood C, Kontopantelis E, Reeves D. Effect of financial incentives on inequalities in the delivery of primary clinical care in England: Analysis of clinical activity indicators for the quality and outcomes framework. Lancet. 2008 Aug 30;372(9640):728–736.

97. American Medical Group Association. High-performing health system definition. Alexandria, VA: American Medical Group Association. 2013 [cited August 20, 2013]. As of November 5, 2013:
http://www.amga.org/Advocacy/HPHS/hphsDefinitionHandout.pdf

98. Beich J, Scanlon DP, Ulbrecht J, Ford EW, Ibrahim IA. The role of disease management in pay-for-performance programs for improving the care of chronically ill patients. Medical Care Research and Review. 2006 Feb;63(1 Suppl):96S–116S.

99. Conrad DA, Christianson JB. Penetrating the "black box": financial incentives for enhancing the quality of physician services. Medical Care Research and Review. 2004 Sep;61(3 Suppl):37S-68S.

100. Frolich A, Talavera JA, Broadhead P, Dudley RA. A behavioral model of clinician responses to incentives to improve quality. Health Policy. 2007 Jan;80(1):179–193.

101. Rosenthal MB, Frank RG. What is the empirical basis for paying for quality in health care? Medical Care Research and Review. 2006 Apr;63(2):135–157.

102. Vina ER, Rhew DC, Weingarten SR, Weingarten JB, Chang JT. Relationship between organizational factors and performance among pay-for-performance hospitals. Journal of General Internal Medicine. 2009 Jul;24(7):833–840.

103. Yale New Haven Health Services Corporation. Medicare Hospital Quality Chartbook: Performance Report on Outcome Measures. Baltimore, MD: Centers for Medicare and Medicaid Services. 2012.

104. Lake TK, Stewart KA, Ginsburg PB. Lessons from the field making accountable care organizations real. [Book; Computer File; Internet Resource Date of Entry: 20110708]: Washington, D.C. : Center for Studying Health System Change. 2011 [cited 2011 July 8]; 7, [1] p. : digital, PDF file, ill.].

105. Moore K, Coddington D. From Volume to Value: the Transition to Accountable Care Organizations. Greenwood Village: McCannis Consulting. 2011.

106. Shields MC, Patel PH, Manning M, Sacks L. A model for integrating independent physicians into accountable care organizations. Health Affairs. 2011 Jan;30(1):161–172.

107. Shortell SM, Casalino LP. Implementing qualifications criteria and technical assistance for accountable care organizations. JAMA. 2010 May 5;303(17):1747–1748.

108. Chung S, Palaniappan L, Wong E, Rubin H, Luft H. Does the frequency of pay-for-performance payment matter?—Experience from a randomized trial. Health Services Research. 2010 Apr;45(2):553–564.

109. Arling G, Job C, Cooke V. Medicaid nursing home pay for performance: Where do we stand? Gerontologist. 2009 Oct;49(5):587–595.

110. Ragin CC. Redesigning social inquiry: Fuzzy sets and beyond. Chicago and London: University of Chicago Press. 2008.

111. Ragin CC. Using qualitative comparative analysis to study causal complexity. Health Services Research. 1999 Dec;34(5 Pt 2):1225–1239.

112. Winslow R. HMO juggernaut: U.S. Healthcare cuts costs, grows rapidly and irks some doctors. Wall Street Journal. 1994 Sep: A1.